Praise for *From I Do to We Do*

"This book is a breath of fresh air for couples in the trenches of parenting. Weinstein writes with honesty, humor, and hard-won wisdom that makes you feel seen while also giving you a way forward. If you've ever wondered what happened to us, this is the roadmap back to connection."

—**Dr. Morgan Cutlip,**
relationship therapist and author

"*From I Do to We Do* is the kind of book every parent in the trenches of raising kids and keeping a marriage alive needs! With honesty, humor, and heart, Weinstein offers couples both validation and practical tools for staying connected when life feels chaotic. This book is a lifeline for partners who want to thrive, not just survive, in the parenting years."

—**Dr. Cassidy Freitas,**
licensed marriage and family therapist
and host of *Holding Space* podcast

"This book is a must-read is for anyone who knows there's more available in their relationships—more honesty, more connection, more love—and is ready to step into that. Page after page, I felt Weinstein's words jumping out at me, almost as if he were telling my story. I found deep resonance, solace, and hope in this book. If you're willing to be challenged to grow without losing sight of your humanity, Weinstein will meet you there. His wisdom isn't just intellectual, it's embodied, and it changes the way you see yourself and the people you love. . .in all the best ways."

—**Mark Groves,**
human connection specialist,
author of *Liberated Love,*
and founder of Create The Love

"What makes *From I Do to We Do* so powerful is how Eli weaves in stories and examples every couple can see themselves in while grounding it all in his expertise. It's an honest, hopeful reminder that love can thrive even in the busiest, most challenging seasons."

—**Jennifer Chaiken,**
LMFT, and Emmalee Bierly, LMFT,
co-owners of The Therapy Group and
co-hosts of the *ShrinkChicks* podcast

"Eli Weinstein gets it. Marriage changes after kids, and most couples aren't ready for how much. *From I Do to We Do* helps parents rebuild connection and teamwork, because happier couples raise happier children."

—**Dr. Mona Amin,**
pediatrician and creator of PedsDocTalk,
a global platform for parenting and child health education

"Eli Weinstein writes a brilliant depiction of the challenges parents experience while navigating marriage while also raising children. He expertly and eloquently shares advice in a helpful and honest way to help couples go from surviving to thriving. This is a must-read for any couple struggling with the balance between being a parent and a spouse who is looking to reconnect and rebuild their relationship."

—**Dr. Kim Van Dusen,**
LMFT, RPT, and founder of The Parentologist

"As someone who has spent years helping parents navigate the emotional ups and downs of family life, I found this book to be an invaluable guide. It also feels like sitting down with a friend who gets it. We're reminded that partnership and parenthood don't have to be at odds. They can even strengthen each other when approached with honesty and intention. It is a must-read for every parent who's ever wondered, 'What happened to us?'"

—**Dr. Siggie Cohen,**
child development specialist and founder of drsiggie.com

FROM I DO TO WE DO

Navigating Marriage in the Parenting Years

ELI WEINSTEIN, LCSW

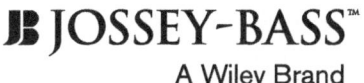

A Wiley Brand

Published by John Wiley & Sons, Inc., Hoboken, New Jersey.

ISBNs: 9781394318698 (Paperback), 9781394318704 (ePub), 9781394318711 (ePDF)

For general information on our other products and services or for technical support, please contact our Customer Care Department within the United States at (800) 762-2974, outside the United States at (317) 572-3993 or fax (317) 572-4002.

Wiley also publishes its books in a variety of electronic formats. Some content that appears in print may not be available in electronic formats. For more information about Wiley products, visit our web site at www.wiley.com.

Library of Congress Cataloging-in-Publication Data:

Cover Design: Wiley
Cover Images: © cglade/Getty Images, © Wirestock/Getty Images, © CSA-Plastock/Getty Images
Author Photo: © Justin Harrison
Printed and bound by CPI Group (UK) Ltd, Croydon, CR0 4YY

C9781394318698_140126

To Ariella, Rikki, and Max—you are my heart, my laughter, and my why. Every page of this book carries pieces of our love, chaos, and the life we're building together.

Contents

Introduction: Love, Chaos, and Everything in Between

"Raising kids is part joy and part guerrilla warfare."

—Ed Asner

MUSIC HAS ALWAYS spoken to me, both in the way my ADHD brain hears the different sounds and harmonies and in the way it conveys emotions and feelings that can't often be described in a normal sentence. Over the past few years, one band that I've really connected with is a group called AJR. One song called "100 Bad Days" really speaks to me and explains parenting so perfectly (whether the band realizes it or not):

> A hundred bad days made a hundred good stories
> A hundred good stories make me interesting at parties
> Yeah, no, I ain't scared of you
> No, I ain't scared of you no more

As parents, we see a lot and experience every emotion, some that we didn't even know existed. Despite some of the overwhelming feelings that these new experiences can create, becoming a parent opens the door to discovering new layers within ourselves and our relationships. Even in the days that feel so low, so draining, so stressful, we can look back at these experiences as either stories that are laugh-out-loud hilarious when we're past them or as pivotal moments in our development.

In 2019, my wife and I were two years into the incredible journey of parenthood, blessed with our beautiful daughter after years of IVF treatment and wanting this life so badly. Those early years were filled with joy, wonder, and a sense of fulfillment that we had never experienced before. It felt as if we were living in a dream, maybe even a nightmare at times. Our little family was doing the best it could, and every moment seemed precious.

But as time went on, something began to change. Beneath the surface of our seemingly "perfect" life, there were tensions brewing that we didn't understand. We were so caught up in the day-to-day demands of parenting that we didn't realize the strain it was putting on our relationship. We were unaware of the cracks that were beginning to form, the unspoken needs, and the unresolved issues that were slowly building up between us.

It was our fifth anniversary, and we had a babysitter, a nice hotel, and something we hadn't had in over a year: uninterrupted time together. It should have been perfect. But instead, it imploded.

I don't remember what we were arguing about, but I remember how painful it felt. My wife and I have never fought harder than on that "wonderful vacation," and we haven't fought that hard since. It was one of those all-out screaming matches that shakes you to your core. It felt like a loss of self, like everything I thought I was holding together just exploded in my face, but at the same time, there was this massive relief that the feelings and thoughts finally came out. There were so many unmet needs from two people who just needed to be heard. As a married man and relationship therapist, that day was an eye-opening experience.

Sometimes it takes a tough wake-up call to help us see what we truly need. For my wife and me, that argument was a turning point.

It shifted everything: how we understood ourselves, how we supported each other, and how we chose to move forward in our relationship.

In those hours of pain, the passion and drive behind this book was created. What started as heartbreak slowly turned into clarity and purpose, a deep desire to make sense of the struggle and offer something meaningful to others walking a similar path.

This book is for any, and every, parent who has been in a battle with themselves, their partner, or their family. This book is for the parents not to lose themselves just because they have built a beautiful family.

This book is for every parent who's ever felt torn between being a partner, a parent, and a person.

It's for the couples who whisper, "What happened to us?"

It's for the parents trying to hold it all together, craving connection, and quietly fighting to be seen.

This book is a lifeline.

A reminder that you're not alone.

That your relationship matters.

And that you don't have to disappear just because you became a parent.

This book isn't going to sugarcoat the experiences of struggle, and instead of turning on each other, this book is about learning how to fight *for* each other. It's a guide to staying connected, grounded, and in love while navigating the daily grind of raising kids so you don't lose yourself or your relationship in the process.

Looking back now, I realize that the fight my wife and I had back then was about the culmination of unaddressed struggles, of communication that had broken down without us even realizing it. In that moment, as uncomfortable as it was, we were talking; we were finally confronting the issues that had been simmering beneath the surface. And while it wasn't our finest moment, it was a necessary one. We finally heard and saw each other in ways we needed.

You've probably heard the saying, "If there's a will, there's a way." But honestly, I think we've all had moments in life where that just doesn't feel true. No matter how much determination or love you have, sometimes you're still stuck, unsure of where to turn. That's why a quote I read recently by psychologist Dr. Mark Goulston really hit home: "If there is a way, then there can be will."[i] Instead of forcing yourself to push through life with blind determination, this flips the narrative. When you've got a clear path forward, that clarity is what fuels your drive, not the other way around.

From the moment I became a parent, I felt lost and confused. Everything felt like it was shifting at once. It's taken me on a ride with more unexpected twists and turns than I ever saw coming. I didn't know where to focus my attention or how to even feel grounded in the madness of my identity, my relationship with my partner, and how I viewed life in general, I felt overwhelmed, lost, and like I was fumbling through every decision I made.

People love to say, "Don't worry; you love your family, you'll figure it out." But love alone isn't a roadmap. It's the fuel, not the GPS. Without some kind of direction, you end up running in circles or getting lost, hoping you don't fall apart along the way. I know, I've been there. Love is essential, but it's not a substitute for clarity, intention, and the tools to navigate this new phase of life.

That's where this book comes in. I wanted to create something for people who feel like I did—lost, confused, and trying to figure out how to balance being a good parent and a good partner.

Parenting is hard.

Relationships are hard.

This isn't going to be a book full of fluff and feel-good sound bites. It's going to be honest, unfiltered, and grounded in the real challenges that parents and partners face every day. My goal is to give you the tools to navigate the storm with purpose and confidence.

So, here's my new mantra: "If there is a way, then there can be will." Once you have a direction, you stop feeling stuck. You stop wasting energy on the wrong things and start focusing on what matters. It isn't about being perfect; it's about being intentional in how you show up for your family and yourself.

Parenting and relationships are messy, no doubt about it. But they don't have to be impossible. The key is to stop relying on love alone and figure out how to turn that love into real, actionable steps. Parenting and relationships aren't things you figure out by accident. They're thoughtful, evolving processes that demand meaning and effort. By accepting this reality, we stop feeling like failures when love isn't enough to solve every problem. Instead, we start looking for the way forward.

When I was a teenager, I was part of a youth group called NCSY. At every major event, someone[i] would read a section of Rudyard Kipling's poem *The Law of the Jungle*:

"For the strength of the Pack is the Wolf, and the strength of the Wolf is the Pack."

At the end, hundreds of people would let out a coordinated wolf howl. At first, I found it bizarre, even cultish. But eventually, I understood: it was about unity. A shared rhythm. A signal that no one stands alone.

This is what the ideal parenting unit needs to embrace. The pack mentality of being individuals that are one mind, one soul, and one goal of making the day as successful, smooth, and productive, no matter what the day throws. Imagine how powerful that howl is for bringing everyone back into the team mindset. It's easy to go off and do your own thing, but that can throw off the whole balance. Sometimes we need a reminder to reconnect and move together.

That's the heart of this book: not to perfect parenting but to strengthen the pack.

So if you're ready to stop winging it and start creating a foundation built on connection and clarity, let's begin.

---

[i]Nachum Zack and Jon Ackerman.

Chapter 1: Two's Company, Three's a Circus: Dives into the messy, hilarious realities of parenting and the lessons hiding in plain sight.

Chapter 2: The Holy Trinity: The Foundation of It All: Where love gets tangled between what we hope for, what we see, and what's really happening. This chapter unpacks how expectations, perceptions, and reality shape our relationships—revealing how those forces collide, confuse, and ultimately create the dynamics that can either pull us apart or bring us closer together.

Chapter 3: Gray Area: Where life stops being "all or nothing" and starts being "a little bit of everything." It's real and often the secret ingredient to staying sane in parenting and partnership— showing how embracing nuance helps couples move beyond rigid black-and-white thinking to create space for understanding, balance, and lasting connection.

Chapter 4: Oxygen Tank: Reframes self-care as essential rather than indulgent, revealing how prioritizing your own needs strengthens both your parenting and your partnership.

Chapter 5: Chaos O'Clock: Where Sleep Dies and Survival Begins: Unpacks the reality of running on fumes—where sleep deprivation and emotional overload collide—and shows how couples can survive, adapt, and stay close in the midst of it all.

Chapter 6: From Dudes to Dads: The Role of Fatherhood: Offers a real-talk look at the inner lives of fathers—unpacking their emotional journeys and what it takes for them to feel truly seen, supported, and whole.

Chapter 7: Mama Magic: Explores the emotional landscape of motherhood, highlighting the needs, challenges, and strengths that help mothers feel recognized, supported, and whole.

Chapter 8: Pillow Talk 2.0:   Explores how honest, attuned communication can strengthen connection and keep couples close—no matter how unpredictable life becomes.

Chapter 9: Love and War: Conflict is inevitable, but disconnection doesn't have to be. Learn how to fight fair, listen with empathy, and repair quickly—turning arguments into opportunities for deeper understanding and lasting closeness.

Chapter 10: Us vs. Them: Covers how to strengthen your team dynamic and parent as a united front—maintaining connection and consistency, even in the face of disagreement.

Chapter 11: The Secret Life of Small Moments: Talks about how to find presence and meaning in the little things—the unnoticed moments that end up meaning everything.

Chapter 12: Rediscovering Us: More Than Just Date Night: Guides couples in rebuilding intimacy and rediscovering their partnership—opening the door to deeper love and lasting connection.

I'm so honored you picked this book up to join me on this wild ride of relationships and parenting. Maybe together we can find a way to thrive in all the ways we have hoped.

Note

1. Goulston, Mark, and Philip Goldberg, *Out of Your Own Way: Overcoming Self-Defeating Behavior* (New York: Perigee, 1996).

1

Two's a Company, Three's a Circus

"You gain strength, courage, and confidence by every experience in which you really stop to look fear in the face."

—Eleanor Roosevelt

THIS IS THE chapter I wished someone had written for me before I had kids. It's raw and as real as it gets. Let's strip away the fluff, the Instagram-perfect family photos, and the sugarcoated "it's all worth it" speeches.

Let's start with the advice I got before having kids. I remember it vividly because it came packaged in these neat little sound bites, always accompanied by a smug grin or a knowing laugh. Here are the greatest hits:

- "Get sleep now because you'll never sleep again."
- "As long as you love them, everything will work out."
- "It only gets better, so know that the beginning is the hardest part."
- "Happy wife, happy life."

Here's the thing about these one-liners: they're well-meaning but wildly unhelpful. Advice givers want to ease your mind, or maybe lighten the mood. But platitudes don't prepare you for the

1

24/7 reality of parenthood. They don't tell you about the sheer exhaustion, the feelings of inadequacy, the guilt that creeps in when you lose your temper, or the quiet relief you feel when daycare or school gives you a break and how that relief makes you question yourself.

Most people are ashamed to speak about the loneliness that sometimes hits when the world is asleep and you're awake with a crying baby or when you feel like you are the only one on this huge planet who is struggling to survive the daily grind. Nobody ever sat me down and said, "Hey, this is going to be the most physically, mentally, and emotionally exhausting thing you've ever done. It'll shake you to your core, but you'll find strength in yourself that you never knew existed."

That would've been the truth; it probably would have sent me into a spiral, but I think I would have appreciated the honesty.

As a therapist, I've spent years learning to listen deeply, read between the lines, and recognize what's left unsaid. And if there's one thing I've learned, it's that your partner may be afraid to tell you the truth. Maybe they think it'll scare you off. Maybe they're worried you'll judge them. But you deserve the truth. You deserve to know what you're walking into. And if it scares you? Good. Fear is healthy; it's your brain trying to prepare you for what's ahead. Let's face what's ahead instead of avoiding it.

Before we dive into the realities of parenting, let's take a moment to rewind and reflect on what came before: your relationship, just the two of you. In those early days, love often feels easy and full of hope. There's time to connect, space to dream, and energy to pour into each other without the constant demands of caregiving. Cue the slow-motion montage and dramatic ballad[i] because back then, everything felt magical, even cinematic. That foundation matters because the connection you build during that phase becomes the anchor when life gets more complex. As a couple, you've been building routines, enjoying freedoms, having time to talk, and

---

[i]Michael Bolton as he serenades our ears with "When a Man Loves a Woman."

maybe even sneaking in weekends away. Yes, there are challenges and conflicts, but there's also an energy of hope and possibility.

I've seen many couples rush past the chance to deepen their bond before becoming parents, missing the opportunity to build the strongest foundation of all, their relationship. That connection is what holds everything together when the chaos of parenting begins. One of the most important things you can do before the baby arrives is invest in your relationship, go on dates, have honest conversations, and talk openly about your hopes, fears, and expectations.

If you're already past that stage, don't panic; we'll be talking in detail in an upcoming chapter about how to strengthen your relationship after the baby arrives. For now, know that once the baby is here, you'll be in survival mode, and even the strongest couples can feel the strain. It's not about love being lost but about learning to navigate a whole new world together so you don't lose sight of each other in the chaos.

All the arguments, compromises, adventures, and joys before kids shift, and in many ways, you have to start from scratch. As therapist Dr. John Delony said, when the baby comes, all that history is dead; it's time to rebuild a new version of the relationship—one that can withstand the realities you're about to face.

And that brings us to the heart of it—parenting isn't just about diapers and midnight feedings; it's about doing all of that while trying to keep your relationship (and your sanity) intact. That is where the real, messy, hilarious, and sometimes downright absurd moments begin.

Obviously, parenting isn't all torturous and demonic experiences, but it is one of the biggest challenges that pushes you in directions you never knew you could go. There is something amazing that happens: you learn your way of rolling with the punches as a parent and know how to handle what might come your way in the future.

I have told this story often, but when we had our first kid (Rikki), she slept so well at night, giving us four to five hours at a time. We felt so drained by that, going from 8 to 10 hours, and we had no idea how blessed we were. We felt we had all the parenting stuff down, and we did, for her. Then we had Max, and he flipped the script on us, sleeping only one to two hours at a time. But by that time, my wife and I had so many conversations about how we as individuals need to show up for each other, that yes, it was difficult, but we handled it a lot better than we did with Rikki that was an "easier" time.

I spoke with a new mom and dad a few years ago, and here was a breakdown of their conversation four to six months into having a newborn. We'll call them Olivia and Eric:

Eric: *I am trying so hard to connect and be back to where we were before the baby, but she won't even look at me in the morning or say hi to me.*

Olivia: *Yeah...cuz I can't stand your damn breathing...have you noticed how loud it is...I just want to rip your mouth off because it bugs me so much.*

Eric: *Seriously? My breathing is too much, what the hell does that even mean?*

Olivia: *You just don't get it...and that bugs me even more.*

Next argument:

Olivia: *I was trying to be sexy for him this week, be playful and fun...I even grabbed his butt and kissed him on the neck the way he likes. AND I made him his favorite dish. Do you know how tired I am? What do I get? Not even a thank-you.*

Eric: *I didn't know you needed to be thanked for kissing your husband or making food for the family. When did you get so needy?*

Olivia: *Are you serious?! After all I have been doing—that's the way you are talking to me?*

Eric: *I just don't understand what you want from me.*

Another argument:

Eric: *Seriously, another dirty diaper...what are we feeding this kid!*

Olivia: *Stop complaining; I've changed 12 today.*

Eric: *I wasn't complaining at all; I am just shocked by the amount of poop our kid has.*

Olivia: Well, it sounded like you were criticizing how I was feeding her. I'm doing my best.

Eric: What?! I know you are. How did we get to this being about you? I was just stating a fact about our kid and all the diapers we have to change.

Olivia: I don't know. Just get her into the bath and change her after...I got it. Thanks.

Throughout all these arguments, there is a clear disconnect and struggle to hear each other's genuine concerns and pains, because in the moment it's all about survival. What could have prepared them for struggles and arguments like this? Did this couple ever imagine they'd be arguing about breathing or poop volumes?

As I wrote in the introduction, this was what my first year of having my daughter was like: constant bickering and being at each other's throats for nothing big and everything small. This doesn't have to be the norm for couples who have kids.

What is normal:

- Being stressed
- Being tired
- Being uncertain and overwhelmed
- Learning on the go
- Pivoting and adjusting to what the day throws at you

Parenthood is like stepping into a world like the Upside Down in *Stranger Things*, where life is similar but off enough that you notice. Suddenly, you're not just you anymore; you're someone's mom or dad, a title that comes with a whole new set of responsibilities and emotions and a lot less sleep and more crying, and not just from the baby. It's one of the most profound transformations a person can experience. While it's filled with moments of pure joy and love, it's also a journey that can leave you questioning, "Wait, who am I again?" and "Why did we want to do this?" and, as I have felt lately, "Can I revoke my adult membership card?"

These questions are so important to ask, and more importantly we need to be kind to ourselves when we ask them.

Parenthood is an incredible journey, one that reshapes every aspect of your life, including your sense of self, and I wouldn't change it for the world. I wanted to share some stories I have had over the years that truly enlighten parents and couples to the realities of having kids and the many magical ways they can add to your life.

When Poop Does Hit the Fan

Years ago, it was time to spend some of the Jewish holidays with my family. After just a few months of becoming new parents, we lacked crucial knowledge of the random things that can, could, and will happen as parents. We had no idea how to pack, how to travel, or even what we needed for our own home for our kid, let alone someone else's home.

For this trip, we were sleeping in the same room as our daughter. Who knew such a little person could make so many noises in the night?[ii] This is what it feels like when you have a newborn. You're exhausted, barely awake, and still expected to function. And if you're not quiet enough, the baby wakes up, and then you're stuck for hours with a newborn ready to party.

My daughter decided to wake up while we were sleeping. As a new parent, you are taught to go through a basic checklist of what could be wrong:

- Dirty diaper
- Gas bubble
- Hunger

So, we started with the first option and were surprised by something that made us scream and jump out of the way. We both got up to help since at that time, I felt like a disconnected third wheel in

---

[ii] I always make this joke about a new competition game I want to create. Let's stop with all these quiz games that test people's knowledge or being able to remember random facts, but instead sleep deprive the contestants for two to three days and ask them to be woken up abruptly and do basic tasks in half-lit rooms and see who wins. That's true skill.

the family, so this was my way of playing a role in being a part of my kid's life. It was dark, and we didn't want to wake the baby, hoping we could quickly solve the problem and get back to bed. Well, my daughter had other plans and decided to let out a massive shart that shot across the room at us. We both yelled, jumped out of the way, and scared her all at the same time. We were so shaken up and didn't even process how funny the situation was till the morning when we could see the range, damage, and amount of poop that got all over a white carpet in the room we were sleeping in. We laughed about it, and now it's a hilarious story because poop literally hit the fan!

A lot of times you will go through what seems to be such stressful and "traumatic" moments as a parent and we lose sight of the silliness and ridiculousness that raising kids can bring. Please don't lose sight of opening your heart to laughter and having some humor, even dark humor, to get through the hard times that happen in the adventures of daily life with little gremlins.

Figuring It Out

Parenting reminds me of one of my favorite scenes from *Daddy Day Care*. There's a little boy who's struggling with potty training and wants to prove he can handle going to the bathroom on his own, like a "big boy." Eddie Murphy's character steps in to check on him, and what he finds is absolute chaos, a bathroom destroyed. His reaction, a mix of shock, disbelief, and "How is this even possible?" is hilarious and unforgettable.

That scene captures the reality of parenting. Kids are messy and unpredictable and often leave you wondering how such a small person could cause so much destruction. Whether it's a bathroom disaster, the number of toys they "have" to play with by throwing them all over the room, spilled cereal on the floor, or crayon marks on the walls, there are moments that leave you shaking your head, trying not to laugh and cry at the same time.

When I first started as a therapist, I was thrown into the deep end—working at a clinic and seeing more than 40 clients a week.

If this were a therapy book, those two years would warrant a whole chapter on how unsustainable that workload was. But that's a story for my second book.

For now, I want to zoom in on one night that's stuck with me ever since.

Back then, I worked two nights a week until 10 p.m. because weekend shifts weren't an option—I observe the Sabbath. One of those nights, as I was wrapping up a session and prepping for the next, my phone buzzed. It was my wife, panicked.

She had been giving our daughter a bath when things took a turn: a full-blown poop explosion. Not a little mess—a "How is this physically possible?" kind of mess. She was overwhelmed, trying to figure out how to contain it, clean it, and not lose her mind.

She needed backup. Fast.

But I couldn't leave. I had clients stacked back-to-back for the rest of the night, and there was no way out. All I could do was apologize over the phone, feeling helpless and consumed by guilt. She was knee-deep in chaos, and I was stuck in my tiny office, counting the minutes until I could get home.

There's a humbling kind of magic in parenting: even in the most chaotic, poop-filled disasters, you somehow figure it out. It's never perfect, it's exhausting and sometimes ridiculous, but you manage to get it done. This was one of those moments for my wife.

Overwhelmed but determined, she sprang into action. With a roll of paper towels, she wrapped our daughter like a tiny burrito and placed her safely on the floor. Then she tackled the war zone that was the tub—draining, scrubbing, and sanitizing like a pro. When it was finally clean, she realized a second bath wasn't in the cards. So she improvised.

She cleared the dishes (yes, she thought of that!) and gave our daughter a bath in the kitchen sink.

It wasn't glamorous, but it worked. By the time I got home, they were both squeaky clean—and somehow half-laughing about the whole thing.

Moments like this remind you: parenting isn't about perfection. It's about survival, creativity, and making it work—one messy, chaotic step at a time.

It taught me a massive lesson. We need to learn to be flexible and resourceful or parenting will crush us in ways we never imagined. But with each challenge, poop explosion, tantrum, and terrible car ride, we learn to adapt. For some, the strength to handle it comes naturally. For others, it grows with time, practice, and those unexpected moments that call us to rise. Sure, the stress can feel like you're drowning, but somehow you find ways to crawl through. It's rarely graceful, maybe even covered in vomit and poop, but it gets done, and we are so much stronger afterward.

Find Your Way

When I was growing up, I remember we had a random house guest over the weekend. They brought their very cute son with them and spent the weekend with us. There is a vivid moment from the whole weekend that stuck out to me.

The son was struggling to adjust to the new space, as it was outside his comfort zone, and his parents were finding it tough to get him to calm down. They went to my parents and asked if we had a handheld vacuum. With a confused expression, my mom said we didn't, and the parents looked dismayed. Then the dad screamed with excitement that he had his shaver. He ran into the other room and began running it near the baby. Within minutes, the kid calmed down.

I remember this because it seemed insane at the time; who the heck calms their kid down with a shaver or a vacuum? Parents do. All parents have their way of doing things that have worked a few times, and they put it in the bank of their mind as random things to do as a way to calm their screaming child. For these parents, it was the humming noise of a vacuum or shaver, so wherever they went, they had one handy at all times.

In the beginning, our daughter was a decent sleeper, giving us blissful four- to five-hour stretches. But getting her *to* sleep? That was a whole production.

Like many parents (no judgment here), we had our own oddly specific routine. For us, it meant holding her at a twisted angle while bouncing our knees in just the right rhythm. We did it so long some nights that my arms would go numb. From the outside, it probably looked like we were giving her a low-budget rollercoaster ride—but it worked.

I remember once at a family meal, my sister-in-law offered to soothe her. She did what any normal person would do: a gentle, classic rock. But nope, that didn't cut it. We had to jump in and teach her "the move," because anything less wouldn't do.

Every parent has their own way, whether it's feeding, bathing, dressing, or bedtime routines. So let's all do each other a favor: stop judging.

What works for one kid—or one stage—might not work for another. That's the reality. This is especially for the friends, grandparents, aunts, uncles, and anyone else in the village helping raise these little ones: *don't question or push back in the moment.* Respect the parents' choices. If you're curious, ask later—gently and without judgment.

Of course, safety always comes first. Abuse or harm can never be excused as a "parenting style." But when it comes to the everyday stuff—how we keep our kids content and ourselves from falling apart—parents need space to figure it out.

Give yourself the freedom to get creative. Don't let criticism, social media "experts," or one failed attempt shake your confidence. Be patient. You'll find what works best for you and your family.

Parenting constantly teaches, whether you're ready to learn or not. Between my own experiences and stories from clients, I've heard it all. Some make me laugh, some still bring me to tears, and others just leave me stunned at the absurdity. But one thing is certain: parenting brings out both the best and the most challenging parts of who we are.

Let me start with this: I'm not coming to you as someone who has it all figured out. I'm not a perfect parent, and I've yet to meet anyone who is. What I do have is perspective. Between my own parenting journey and the countless families I've worked with, I've seen what helps, what hurts, and—most importantly—how to find what actually works for you.

My goal isn't to tell you what to do but to give you the tools you need to strengthen your relationships and navigate the hard moments.

Parenting is not a cakewalk. It's draining, and sometimes it feels impossible. But you are capable. You are strong enough to handle this. Even when you're running on fumes and feel like you're failing, you are still doing something remarkable. The very act of showing up, day after day, is enough to prove that you've got what it takes. You're not alone, and you don't have to figure it out all by yourself.

Throughout this book, I'll be walking alongside you. We'll face some of the hardest parts of parenting, the moments that feel impossible, the cracks that may have formed in your relationship with your partner, or even within yourself. Together, we'll explore how to repair what's been strained, strengthen what's still standing, and rediscover the joy that often gets buried beneath the daily grind.

As we move forward, remember: parenting isn't just about your kids; it's about *you*, too. It's about who you are, how you show up, and how you manage the expectations you place on yourself and others.

That brings us to a core concept I call the "Holy Trinity" of parenting: *expectations, perceptions,* and *reality.* These three forces are constantly in motion, shaping how we experience ourselves, our relationships, and the journey we're on.

In the next chapter, we're going to dive into this "Holy Trinity." We'll talk about the trap of expectations, including the ones we place on ourselves, the ones society places on us, and the ones we impose on our children. We'll examine how our perceptions of what parenting should look like often clash with the imperfect reality. Most importantly, we'll figure out how to let go of what isn't serving us so we can focus on what truly matters.

So, take a deep breath. You've made it this far, and that's no small thing. Let's keep going together, one story, one lesson, one step at a time.

As Theodore Roosevelt said, "When you're at the end of your rope, tie a knot and hold on."

2

The Holy Trinity: The Foundation of It All

"I'm not in this world to live up to your expectations, and you're not in this world to live up to mine."

—Bruce Lee

WHEN MY DAUGHTER was born, I was fortunate to have a job that offered 12 weeks of paternity leave through New York Paid Family Leave. I was genuinely excited about this time with her. After years of infertility and a frightening emergency C-section, our daughter felt like the biggest miracle, and I couldn't wait to spend those precious weeks bonding with her.

My wife had already spent nine weeks at home with our daughter, not only recovering from emergency surgery but also breastfeeding, pumping, and doing her best to keep the household running. She was exhausted but had kept everything afloat. When it was finally my turn to take over, I imagined peaceful days of cuddling and bonding. What I didn't anticipate was just how demanding full-time baby care would be. I felt completely unprepared for what caring full-time for a newborn actually entailed. All my fears and worries crept in that I would totally mess up this opportunity of connection that I desperately needed with my daughter.

Quickly I realized that being home all day with a baby who refused to nap wasn't as glamorous as I had envisioned. The days blurred into an endless cycle of feeding, changing, and cleaning up after a newborn, all while attempting to keep the house somewhat presentable. Meanwhile, my wife's transition back to work was anything but easy. Her day started at 4:30 a.m., nursing our daughter, putting her back down, getting herself ready, preparing all of her pumping materials, commuting an hour each way, pumping during whatever breaks she could find, working a full day, and then making the exhausting journey home.

One evening, when my wife walked through the door, she took one look around at the mess surrounding me and our daughter. In that instant, I saw a look on her face that I interpreted as: *Seriously? This is what I'm coming home to? What have you been doing all day?*

I felt a depth of judgment and shame in that moment that I never experienced, like all my efforts with our daughter were nothing, and the only focus was on the things I didn't do.

We all have likely felt this feeling internally about our partners at least once (or 20) times a day, but this was the first time it pierced my heart with as much power to crush my soul. But the truth was, we were both exhausted in different ways, both adjusting to new challenges neither of us had fully anticipated. That moment wasn't about judgment; it was a sign that we needed to communicate better, to align our expectations with reality, and to support each other as partners in this new phase of our lives.

This is when the thought process of the *Holy Trinity* was created. I began to see it everywhere with my clients, especially married couples with kids. The idea is that in her mind she expected more to be done, and I knew that there was nothing more I could do, but she had no idea about what actually went down:

- Changing diapers
- Rocking my daughter to sleep (for longer than hoped but oh so yummy)
- Cleaning bottles
- Warming bottles
- Cleaning more bottles

- Cleaning up a poop explosion
- Changing another diaper
- Rocking her again!
- Being spit up on/pooped on
- Feeding her again
- Getting spit up on again!

But all she saw was a messy house and me sitting and waiting for her to come home with the baby sleeping on my chest.

Don't get me wrong, I loved most of the experience of paternity leave (I'll get into it more in Chapter 5), but I was doing all I could, and all I felt was failure in that one look and moment.

The Holy Trinity refers to three fundamental components of life and thought process in everyday experiences: *expectations*, *perceptions*, and *realities*.

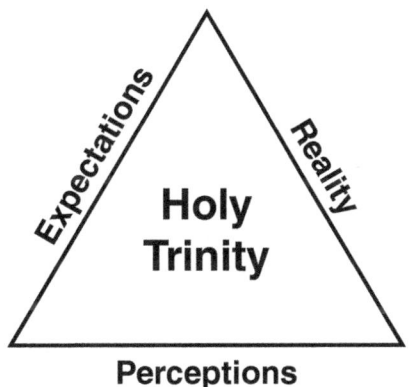

Understanding this trio has become one of the most important insights I return to both in my own life and in my work with couples. How we experience and navigate our roles as parents and partners can be defined by the understanding and work on the trio we're about to dive into.

In almost 10 years of being a therapist, I've noticed how easy it is to get stuck in one part of the triangle. When we can't accept or move forward, it quietly chips away at our relationships—building up resentment and painful thoughts toward the people we love, often without them even knowing it. These bumps and stops in the flow of our thought process can stop us from connecting or even wanting to be around our partners due to disgust or annoyance and can derail a wonderful relationship from growing, even causing it to end.

Let's start explaining this concept and how we can apply it to our daily lives and then build up to what this book is all about, our relationship with our partner.

- **Expectations:** These are the outlooks we carry around like a heavy backpack, stuffed with ideas about how things *should* be. They're usually packed by our culture, our families, our own wild experiences, and, of course, society's endless stream of "helpful" advice. I'm looking at you social media "experts."
- **Perceptions:** Perceptions are those funky glasses we all wear. They are the invisible ones that color how we see and make sense of everything around us. They're shaped by our brain's quirks, our day-to-day emotions, and our past lived experiences.
- **Realities:** Reality is what's really going on, whether we like it or not, totally ignoring our wishful thinking and rose-colored glasses. It's the cold, hard truth, though we often see it through our own, sometimes foggy, lenses.

The dance between our expectations, perceptions, and reality can either make things flow smoothly or turn into a chaotic mess in relationships and parenting. When these three are in sync, life feels pretty good, and we're all singing the same tune. But when they're out of whack, it's like trying to waltz while everyone else is dancing to a completely different rhythm.

Over the years of working with couples, I have noticed that many people don't have hard conversations about their expectations of love and marriage, as well as how they want to raise a family and parent their kids. Most of the conversations stay at the surface level, which feels comfortable and keeps the relationship moving forward. But eventually, unspoken expectations start to show up, and that's usually when I get called in. My job is to help couples identify those issues, clarify what they really want, and work toward moving forward, ideally together.

A couple of years ago, I worked with a pair named Alani and Cooper. Alani grew up in an immigrant household where the environment was intense—centered around academics, achievement, and proper behavior. Cooper, on the other hand, was raised in a middle-class American family that also valued education but placed a greater emphasis on emotions, family time, and the effort behind hard work rather than the outcome.

Let me be clear, neither upbringing was "wrong." That's not the point of this example. What this illustrates is something I see often: two people coming into a relationship with very different backgrounds and belief systems. In this case, Alani and Cooper initially sought help because they were clashing over how to raise their son. But as we dug deeper, the work naturally expanded to include their relationship, not just their parenting.

Three of the major disagreements they had were over where to send their kid to school, mealtime/playtime style, and religious practices.

School

Alani: *I want my kids to go to private school; it is the only way to set them up for success in their future. If we don't set the foundation now, they will never get into Yale, Harvard, or Columbia, and they will never be successful.*

Cooper: *Really? I went to public school and I am pretty successful. What are you saying about me? And can we talk through this instead of you deciding it and not including me? This is going to cost us so much, and who knows if it's even the "right" option for our kid and family?*

Mealtime

Cooper: *I grew up in a home where we sat together as a family and connected over the dinner table. It means the world to me to have these moments with my kids and wife and create memories every day of our lives together.*

Alani: *Who cares? I just want my son to eat, and if it means distracting him with an iPad at the table, then that's all that matters. We can talk, and he can eat.*

Cooper: *But we don't even talk because you are so hyper-focused on shoving food into his face; you can't even stop for a moment to talk about work, your day or us. It's like I don't even matter.*

Religious Practices

Cooper: *You don't want to circumcise our son! It's one of the most important things in my religion, and I am hearing about this now? I am so in shock and outraged that you aren't on board with this, quoting some "scientist" with no credentials and doctors who aren't religious say it's better for hygiene.*

Alani: *No one is going to mutilate my baby, ever! And my scientist isn't stupid! I looked into it, and I don't want that for my son, ever!*

What shocked me most was how little they had communicated their expectations throughout years of dating, marriage, and even raising their five-year-old. These unspoken assumptions built up over time, leading to confusion, resentment, and emotional disconnection—eventually bringing them into my office.

Instead of addressing the real issue, they kept circling around surface-level needs and wants. It became a cycle of *"Me! Me! Me!"*—with little room for the other person's reality, truth, or emotional experience. When we enter a situation with our minds already made up, we leave no room for other ideas or perspectives. This can do a real disservice to the shared reality we're trying to build especially with the partner we chose to raise a family with. They weren't wrong for having needs. But without mutual understanding or vulnerability, their dynamic became more about competing perspectives than shared growth.

Now let's explore how expectations are shaped and how we can push back against outside pressures. The goal is to create more inner peace, so we can express our needs and positively shape our reality.

Expectations: What No One Says Out Loud

Expectations are like those unwritten rules that everyone seems to know about, yet nobody really talks about until they're not met. Suddenly, it's like you're playing a game with invisible rules, and you're the only one who didn't get the memo. If we don't take the time to understand where they come from and how they're formed, they can lead us straight into a whirlwind of misunderstanding and conflict.

There is a very interesting phenomenon called *naïve realism*[1] coined by Bertrand Russel. This is the tendency to think that the way you see the world is the way it really is, without realizing your perspective might be influenced by your own biases or experiences. Who doesn't feel they have the "right" view on things, especially when it comes to parenting and your relationship? We get tunnel vision of how the world needs to be for there to be success and happiness.

According to Jonathan Haidt's 2006 book, *The Happiness Hypothesis*, this is the biggest obstacle to social harmony in our world. When we view our perspective as the only truth and do not allow our minds to open to other realities, we are stealing our world of beauty and connection.

There are three main factors that can influence our expectations:

- Culture/religion
- Friends, family, and social media
- Personal experiences

Culture/Religion

I want to address this with sensitivity and kindness. As someone who grew up in a religious home as an orthodox Jew and still a very active member of that community, I am not here to bash any religious or cultural beliefs. I am just here to shed light on how they can impact the way we view parenting and relationships and shape us in ways we sometimes aren't aware of.

Picture this: you're a new parent, and suddenly, everyone around you seems to have an opinion on how you should raise your kids. From the type of diapers you use to how you feed your baby and from the rituals you choose—whether baptism, circumcision, or another rite of passage—to the ways you decide to educate your kids, every choice carries meaning and weight, there's no shortage of (mostly) unsolicited advice.

A lot of these expectations are rooted in cultural norms, those ingrained beliefs about what a "good" parent looks like. Maybe your culture emphasizes the father as the main breadwinner while the mother stays home with the kids. Or perhaps it's the other way around. Either way, these cultural blueprints can shape the expectations you have for yourself and your partner, sometimes without you even realizing it.

What was done back in the old country, or the way your grandparents (or even parents) used to do it, might not work for you or translate to today's world. But I have seen for myself, and with many people I have worked with over the years, a very intense guilt and internal battle to respect their heritage, culture, and family belief system. It's a tough balance trying to build your own life while still carrying pieces of your past and looking ahead to the future.

Myles: *I grew up in such an intense environment of guilt and doing better for God that it filled me with so much fear and anxiety. I decided a long time ago that I wouldn't live that life and wouldn't raise my kids within that. My family feels that I am screwing up my kids because I don't want to put that pressure on them to perform and be something I don't believe in anymore.*

Khloe: *Growing up, there was one option: your kid gets baptized no matter what. That's all I knew, and honestly, I didn't know any kid who didn't get baptized. It is such an integral part of my thought process and a given that being something my wife would be OK with, so I never discussed it. Well now that we have our first kid, she doesn't believe in it at all, and it's breaking my soul. I can't sleep, and I can't look my family in the eyes and let them know it won't be happening...I'm in total shock.*

These stories aren't about judging what's right or wrong—they're about the weight we carry from the worlds we come from. Culture and religion can give us a deep sense of belonging, but they can also create friction when we haven't talked about what they mean to us now. The goal isn't to throw away where we came from. It's about recognizing how those roots shape us, enabling us to have more honest conversations, make choices we both believe in, and build a family that feels true to who we are today.

Friends, Family, and Social Media

The original source code of our expectations. The way we saw our parents handle their relationship and parenting duties tends to set the stage for what we think is "normal." If you grew up in a house where one parent was the emotional rock and the other was the silent provider, you might expect to fall into similar roles in your own family. Or, if emotions were never openly discussed at home, you might unconsciously expect your partner to deal with stress quietly, just like your parents did. But here's the kicker: those expectations might not align with your partner's experience, leading to all kinds of fun surprises.

Over the last few years, I have worked with a few clients on the idea of family shaping our expectations and the way it impacts our relationships and parenting:

Selena: *Growing up, you sacrificed for your kids and family, no questions asked. To me, this is such a powerful lesson to be able to show up for your family. With my wife's family, all they do is talk smack, make fun of, and disrespect each other, and it makes my skin crawl. I feel like they talk badly about me behind my back, and I would never do that to them. I feel no sense of respect for my needs, wants, and beliefs, and I feel so lonely when I am around my wife's family. It causes so many hard and hurtful arguments between how often we spend with his family versus my family, and it impacts my mood and outlook associated with all things his family. It really pains me.*

Lilly: *I grew up in a home that was filled with love and showing up for my kids, no matter what. And that is how I want to show up for my kids and wife. But my wife's family was raised differently, and I just don't understand it. They are more selfish and don't show up for their kids in the way that I would. They wouldn't show up to a holiday dinner if it wasn't perfectly worked around their lives. In my family, you just show up. It makes me so angry how they think and deal with my wife and my outlook on life.*

Don't get me started on the negative influence social media has had on our lives as parents. Too many people rely on these outlets as expert advice and truth sayers, which can cause such internal pain and judgment of ourselves on the way we parent and show up for our partner.

The feeling I have after scrolling for too long is an emptiness, filled with a whisper of "You are not enough," leaving me with pain about myself and life.

I remember during COVID, there were so many reels and videos of all the "amazing" parents making escape rooms, American Ninja Warrior backyards, or whatever out-of-this-world things for their kids who were trapped inside for far too long. Working with people during that time, I got to see the everyday parent struggle even to get dressed, let alone make an extravagant DIY project. And it left a lot of people feeling judgmental of themselves. Don't get me wrong; share what you want and enjoy your life. But as a viewer, it's easy to see vacations, fancy experiences, and perfect date nights and start comparing yourself to people you don't even know or who are in a totally different stage of life.

You are enough by just showing up. Don't let others define how you are doing.

Even now, as I write this book—something I've poured my heart into—I get comments like, "You're crushing it," or "Must be nice to be raking it in!" And while I know those words aren't meant to hurt, they reflect a disconnect. People see the highlight reel (social media posts, podcast clips, smiling pictures with my kids) and assume I've got it all figured out.

I struggle like everyone else. Our finances are tight, and life's realities kick me down. Social media is what I *want* you to see, but it's not what is actually happening. But no one sees that unless they're in my inner circle. That's the danger of assumption, when we fill in the blanks with someone else's carefully curated version of reality and then hold our own lives up to that illusion.

We are all doing our best and we need to accept that we have limitations. We should stop setting ourselves up with superhuman expectations of life that, in the end, cause us to feel like failures, especially when it comes to our parenting, relationships, and home life.

Parenting Expectation Trap

Now let's dive into some of the common expectations we juggle in relationships and parenting.

In relationships, expectations often revolve around roles, responsibilities, and emotional support. For example, you might expect that household chores should be split 50/50 or that your partner should always be emotionally available whenever you need to vent about your day. Sounds reasonable, right? But when those expectations aren't met, it can leave you feeling resentful, unseen, or wondering if you're the only one doing the heavy lifting.

Parenting expectations can be just as tricky. Maybe you've got this picture in your head of how your kids should behave, such as always polite or never throwing tantrums in the grocery store. Or maybe you expect them to hit every developmental milestone right on time like clockwork or, even better, listen to you when you talk. And let's not forget the expectations you have for yourself as a parent: you should always know what to do, never lose your cool, and never feed them cereal or frozen food for dinner. When these expectations don't match up with reality, it's easy to feel like you're failing at this whole parenting thing.

Expectations aren't inherently bad. They can guide us, give us direction, and help us strive for better or close to something more of what we hope our life will be. The trick is to keep them in check and to recognize when they're helpful and when they're just setting us up for disappointment and turning on our own world. By understanding where our expectations come from and being open to adjusting them, we can navigate the beautiful chaos of relationships and parenting with a bit more grace and a lot more positivity.

Perceptions: The Lens We See Through

Personal Experiences

Every relationship you've had and every challenge you've faced has shaped the expectations you carry today. If you've been hurt by disloyalty in the past, you might now expect full transparency from your partner. If insecurity has been a constant companion, you may crave ongoing reassurance—that you're loved, that you're doing enough, that you're not messing it all up. These experiences create a lens through which you view your current relationships, coloring your expectations in ways that can be both helpful and, well, not so helpful.

I had a client a few years ago who had expectations about men. In one session, we were discussing her struggles in her dating life and some of the roadblocks she had with moving forward to build the life she wanted. Here is what she said:

Serena: *All men are disgusting and have one thing in mind. They can never be trusted. So, no matter what you say, Eli, it won't change my mind that when I come on a date, I am going to be very hesitant about the guy's expectations.*

Me: *So how are you going to be able to let someone into your life if you have a wall up before you even meet them?*

Serena: *That's why I'm here! But in truth, I don't know, and I'm not sure you can help me with this because I think all men are the same. Even you, and I trust you with loads. But in the back of my mind, I hear this little voice telling me to be worried and concerned.*

Me: *Why do you believe this about men?*

Serena: *A couple of years ago I had a really bad experience on a few dates that really solidified this in my mind. All the guys wanted to do was have sex with me on the first date and never truly wanted to build a connection. So how can I trust them?*

The Emotional Echo Chamber

When we're stressed or emotionally raw, our perception doesn't just narrow; it has the tendency to get filtered through a personal pain amplifier. That one small interaction, like your partner walking past you without saying hello, doesn't land as "they're preoccupied or busy." Instead, it lands as "they're ignoring me, or I probably did something to make them upset."

Take Ezra and Jordan. Ezra had been juggling work, a teething toddler, and a strained relationship with his own mother. When Jordan came home and forgot to thank him for handling bedtime, he didn't just feel annoyed; he felt invisible. "It's like I'm doing everything and no one even notices," he said. In therapy, we unpacked not just the moment, but the meaning *he assigned to it.*

In emotionally charged states, our minds scan for cues that confirm what we *fear is true*: that we're unloved, alone, or failing. This is *confirmation bias* in action. Our brains aren't trying to torture us; they're trying to keep us safe by predicting danger based on past wounds. But healing starts when we pause to ask: "What's the story I'm telling myself? Is it the only possible story?" Slowing down our interpretation can soften conflict and open space for connection.

Parenting Through a Foggy Lens

Parenting shifts our emotional baseline. You're chronically tired, overstimulated, and under-supported, and then your partner says something like, "Did you mean to leave the bottle out?" and suddenly it feels like a personal attack. Not because of the words themselves, but because of what they *activate* in your current state.

Imagine Brian, a new dad who hadn't slept more than four hours in a row in weeks. When his wife, Melissa, suggested he "be more careful about diaper changes," he exploded. "So I can't do anything right?" It wasn't about the diaper; it was about how maxed out and unseen he felt.

Parenting doesn't just deplete us; it can distort our lens. The key is recognizing when your lens is fogged. Sometimes it's not the words that hurt, it's the exhaustion and self-doubt we've been carrying all day.

Perception in Relationships: Reading Between the Lines

We're meaning-making machines. It's part of being human. But sometimes, the meaning we make says more about our inner world than the other person's intentions. Your partner sighs loudly while loading the dishwasher, and your brain instantly whispers, "They're pissed at me."

Let's look at Kim and Alex. During a particularly tense week, Alex came home and shut the door a little harder than usual. Kim's heart rate spiked. "Are you mad at me?" she asked, already bracing for a fight. But Alex had just had a frustrating day at work and hadn't even realized how he was coming across.

These micro-misreads are what I call *emotional potholes*; they seem small but can do serious damage over time if we keep tripping into them. And most of them stem from *assumptions instead of inquiry*. (I dive into this more in Chapter 9.)

Curiosity is the relational muscle that keeps resentment from building. Try: "You seem tense—rough day?" Instead of: "What did I do now?" It shifts the dynamic from defense to dialogue. Over time, this small habit becomes a buffer against misinterpretation and builds a culture of emotional safety.

The Role of Past Trauma and Conditioning

In a wonderful book by Bruce Perry and Oprah Winfrey,[2] they dive into a lot of concepts of trauma and how it has shaped us and the way we deal with the world around us, asking the key question, "What happened to you?"

They mention that a lot of people come into therapy thinking the goal is to somehow undo the past or erase what happened. You can't just wipe those experiences from your brain and undo what shaped you. Therapy isn't about deleting those old pathways; it's about building new ones. It's like having this old, bumpy dirt road you've always taken because it's what you know and then slowly paving a new, smoother freeway right next to it. The dirt road is still there, but over time, you don't rely on it as much. You've got a better option now.

Our perception is not created in the moment; it's carried in from the past. As Thich Nhat Hanh says in *A Lifetime of Peace*:

"If you look deeply into the palm of your hand, you will see your parents and all generations of your ancestors. All of them are alive in this moment. Each is present in your body. You are the continuation of each of these people."[3]

If you've been hurt, dismissed, or betrayed before, your nervous system is constantly on alert for history to repeat itself. It's not paranoia; it's protection. But that same protective lens can become a barrier when it distorts current reality.

Take Jamal, who grew up with a father who only noticed him to criticize. Now, as an adult, whenever his wife offers gentle suggestions, "Maybe try a different tone with the kids?" he flinches. It feels like failure, not feedback. Not because she's harsh, but because he's still wired to brace for judgment.

Or Dana, who had an ex who ghosted her for days. When her current partner takes a few hours to respond to a text, her brain screams, "Here we go again."

Trauma reshapes the way we see the world, and relationships are often the mirror where that distortion shows up most clearly. The good news is that perception can evolve. When we bring awareness to our past patterns and work to distinguish old pain from present truth, we create room for healing.

Ask yourself: "Is this about now—or then?" That one question can start to loosen trauma's grip and open space for a more accurate, more compassionate view of the person in front of you.

Realities: The Ground We Actually Stand On

In therapy, we spend a lot of time unpacking perception, but let's not forget about reality. Reality doesn't care about how we *wish* things were or what we think *should* be happening. It's just…what *is*. It's where real change and growth actually happen, if we're honest enough to face it.

Welcome to the Mess

Let's drop the illusion: real life doesn't come with a filter. The highlight reel you scroll through is someone else's best 5%, and comparing your real-life chaos to it is a fast track to resentment and shame.

Take Ana, a mom of two who once told me, "I feel like I'm failing because we had cereal for dinner and I forgot about pajama day, again." When we unpacked it, she had spent her day helping her daughter through a meltdown, emailing a teacher, and picking up groceries. She showed up in *all* the ways that mattered. The reality? Her day was full of effort and love.

What Kids Really Need

One dad I worked with, Evan, beat himself up because he worked long hours and couldn't do the elaborate projects his partner organized. But when we asked his son what he loved most, he said, "When Daddy makes silly voices at bedtime." No prep, no script—just that moment, and it meant everything.

Perfection is a myth. Connection is the goal. Kids won't remember the picture-perfect lunches you spend hours laboring over. They'll remember feeling safe in your presence, being listened to, and laughing during bath time. Let that be enough, because it *is*.

Reality Can Be Better Than the Dream If You Let It

Dr. Seuss has been credited with saying, "You know you're in love when you can't fall asleep because reality is finally better than your dreams."

That sounds sweet and it *can* be true, but only if we're willing to actually see the reality in front of us instead of constantly comparing it to some fantasy version we built in our heads.

So many of us carry an image of how things *should* look. The "perfect partner." The "ideal parent." The life milestones, the family vacations, the tidy living room. Take Mia, she used to feel disappointed that her husband wasn't the romantic, sweep-you-off-your-feet type she had pictured. No flowers. No grand gestures. But over time, she noticed something else; he always made sure her car had gas. He kept her favorite snacks stocked. He texted her to check in before her stressful meetings. Was it dramatic? No. But it was consistent, thoughtful, and real. That's love showing up in the everyday.

When we stop chasing the dream and start appreciating reality for what it is, not what it's *supposed* to be, we make room for a deeper kind of happiness. One that's not built on fantasy, but on presence, effort, and truth.

Import/Export List

Before I got married, a wonderful mentor of mine, Rabbi Josh Goller, taught me this powerful way to work with your partner on ways to manage expectations. It's called the Import–Export Activity. Start by setting aside time when you're both calm, relaxed, and free from distractions. Maybe it's during a quiet evening or as part of a casual date night. The goal is to talk about your shared expectations, hopes, and realities for your relationship, your home, and your family. This isn't the time to rehash old arguments or assign blame; it's a safe space to explore what you both want to import into your relationship and what you hope to export. Think of *imports* as the values and traditions you loved growing up and want to carry forward and *exports* as the habits or dynamics you'd prefer to leave behind.

A crucial tip for this exercise: write it all down. Use paper and pencil, keeping it informal and editable. This isn't a rigid set of rules but a living document, a reflection of your evolving values, priorities, and needs. Writing things down not only makes your ideas tangible but also creates a shared reference point you can revisit over time. My wife and I make it a tradition to review ours every anniversary. We check in on how well we've stayed aligned with our intentions and adjust based on how life has shifted, especially now that kids are in the picture. What worked when we were newlyweds definitely needs a tweak or an overhaul as our family grows.

For example, you might decide that yelling or slamming doors (export) has no place in your home because it creates unnecessary tension. On the flip side, you might agree to keep your home open and welcoming to friends and family (import) because connection and community are deeply important to both of you. These conversations allow you to reflect on how your individual backgrounds shaped you and what kind of environment you want to create together.

Maybe one of you grew up in a family where no one ever said, "I love you," and you've realized you want to change that dynamic. Your import could be creating a home filled with verbal affirmations, where "I'm proud of you" and "I love you" are said freely and often. On the flip side, you might want to export the silent treatment as a way of handling conflict, agreeing instead to prioritize open communication even when it's uncomfortable.

Maybe your import is the idea of family dinners as sacred time—no phones, no TV, just sitting down together and connecting. You could export the habit of letting work dominate your evenings by setting boundaries around work emails and calls after a certain time. Perhaps one of you values hospitality and wants your home to be a place where friends and family feel welcome (import), while the other grew up in a household filled with constant chaos and wants to export the expectation of hosting every single weekend.

There are just a few examples that I have on my import/export list:

Import	Export
Having an open home	Slamming doors during arguments
Family time/vacations	Yelling at each other
Once-a-month date nights	Commenting on body or food habits
Dinner with the family	Criticizing each other in front of the kids
Every other Sunday is for family fun	Storming off when upset

Some of these are based on our past in our own homes, other people's homes, or just general things we have heard over the years we want to implement.

The beauty of this process is that it's never set in stone. It's about fostering dialogue and mutual understanding, not creating a set of rules to live by. Life is unpredictable, and your needs, values, and perspectives will change over time. The key is to keep evolving, keep talking, and keep growing together. When something feels off in your relationship or family dynamic, don't hesitate to pull out your blueprint, revisit the conversation, and make adjustments as needed. This exercise becomes a tool for accountability but also for compassion and connection.

At its core, this isn't just about what you write; it's about the act of sitting down together, listening, and being intentional about building a life you both love.

As Epictetus said so powerfully, "Do not seek to have events happen as you want them to, but instead want them to happen as they do happen, and your life will go well."

Getting Stuck in the Maze

A couple of years ago, I fell in love with this amazing therapist Phil Stutz. Let me rephrase: the world fell in love with him after one of his clients, Jonah Hill, made a documentary on his therapist.

He shook up the world with his tools and tricks he had developed over the years being an outstanding therapist who prided himself on productive therapy and getting to the root of the issue.

I want to tap into two of these techniques and ideas to help wrap up the expectation traps we can fall into and ways we can get out of them.

Years ago, I was watching the movie *The Shining*, and it solidified in my mind how much I hate bush mazes and of course people who dress their twins up the exact same way. Most of us haven't been chased by a madman in the winter, running after us with an axe (if you have, please speak with a therapist and work through it...sorry). But we usually don't know what it feels like to be trapped and feel like there is no way out.

When I was about 9 or 10 years old, I had in my mind a very scary and disturbing experience: being trapped.

I went to Universal on a trip and was super excited to try new things, see the sights, and *not* go into a haunted house because I *hate* them (still do, even more because of what I am about to tell you). Well, due to peer pressure, I found myself in a haunted house. Back then, the actors and characters were allowed to grab and touch the guests, and I flipped out. I was running in every direction, screaming my head off to find an exit. I felt lost, I was scared, and I almost peed myself with fear of being stuck in that death trap forever.

I've made it through, but I know how easy it is to get stuck in fear when we feel trapped by life's expectations. It can feel like there's no way out, just failure and disappointment.

Getting Out of the Maze

It's 9:47 p.m. The house is finally quiet. There's a pile of dishes in the sink, your toddler's sock is somehow in the fridge, and your partner just walked past you without making eye contact after an argument about God knows what.

You sit on the couch, exhausted, emotionally wiped, and you start to wonder, *When did things get so tense? Weren't we just laughing in the delivery room six months ago?*

That's the thing about parenting; it sneaks in and takes over, not just your schedule, but your connection, your sense of self, and the way you see your partner. It's easy to lose track of the love under the laundry piles and late-night feeds. All you can see is the intensity, resentment building, and struggles with no hope of anything good or positive.

This is where *active love* comes in. It's not about grand gestures or fixing everything in one conversation. It's about intentionally tapping into the good stuff—the real, beautiful moments you've built together—and letting that be your emotional anchor before you spiral or shut down.

Tool #1:

Take a moment to close your eyes or settle into a calm, comfortable space. Picture the good you and your partner have done together—the shared laughs, the quiet triumphs, the moments of connection as you raise your child or children. Let yourself feel the warmth of those memories, and hold that feeling in your heart.

Now, pause and gently check in with yourself: what do you truly need in this moment? Not just what you wish for, but what's real, present, and within reach? When you focus on that, the pressure starts to ease. The impossible standards begin to fade. And in their place, you may find a little more freedom, a little more grounding, and a deeper sense of peace.

Facing the Shadow: Meeting the Parts We Try to Hide

We all carry a shadow. And no, I'm not talking about Darth Vader lurking in the hallway with heavy breathing and unresolved father issues. I'm talking about the parts of ourselves we bury deep, the fears, the shame, the regrets, the harsh self-talk we'd never dare say out loud.

Carl Jung described the shadow as everything we repress or deny. These aren't just "bad" parts; they're often very human emotions we were taught were unacceptable: anger, self-doubt, neediness, even sadness. Left unacknowledged, they fester. They gain power. And without realizing it, we start living *from* our shadow, reacting instead of responding, lashing out instead of leaning in.

In *Inside Out 2*, there's a scene that hit me square in the gut. Riley, the main character, has a locked vault where a deep secret is hidden with her repressed emotions, something she's ashamed of and has been hiding even from herself. When the vault opens, what do we find? A memory of her accidentally burning the rug as a little kid.

That's it.

Not murder. Not betrayal. Just a mistake. A moment. But in her mind, it grew into something monstrous. That's exactly how our shadows work. We hide our regrets and fears so well that we even forget what's in there until the vault bursts open at the worst time. And like Riley, what we've buried often isn't the end of the world; it's the story we've told ourselves *about* it that makes it so painful.

Much like in *Star Wars*, the dark side draws its power from fear and pain. True healing doesn't come from avoiding our shadow; it comes from facing it, understanding it, and integrating it into our whole self. That's the essence of shadow work: acknowledging the parts we tend to hide and transforming them into sources of growth and strength.

Tool #2: Shadow Exercise

Step 1: Sit with yourself. Find a quiet space. Breathe. Grab a notebook or open your Notes app. This is your space; no judgment, just honesty.

Step 2: Write out your shadow. What are the fears, failures, or beliefs you carry about yourself especially around parenting, partnership, or your sense of self?

- *I'm not a good enough dad.*
- *I'm failing my partner.*
- *I'm too much. Or not enough.*

> *Let them out. You're opening the vault—not to live in the past but to understand it.*
>
> **Step 3: Name your shadow.** *Yes, actually name it. Mine changes; sometimes it's Brad. Sometimes Pearl or Petunia. Giving it a name reminds you that your shadow is a part of you, not the whole story.*
>
> **Step 4: Ask it what it wants.** *Every shadow has a purpose; it's usually trying to protect you, just in a twisted way. Ask, "What are you afraid will happen if I don't listen to you? What do you need to feel safe?"*
>
> **Step 5: Let the light in.** *Now write down who you are when you're grounded in truth, not fear.*
>
> - *I'm not perfect, but I'm present.*
> - *I love fiercely, even when I'm tired.*
> - *I'm learning, and that's enough.*
>
> *This is your light. This is your Jedi path. Tape it to your mirror, set it as your lock screen, or read it every time the dark side tries to pull you in.*

Remember, we all have shadows. But the more we ignore them, the more they run the show. When we face them head-on, with curiosity and not shame, we take back the director's chair instead of just following cues.

You're not broken for having dark thoughts. You're human. And healing starts when you say, "I see you" to the shadow and choose light anyway.

As the great and powerful Dumbledore said, "Happiness can be found, even in the darkest of times, if one only remembers to turn on the light."[4]

Understanding how our expectations, realities, and perceptions influence each other is a big step toward building healthier relationships. It means recognizing that our expectations have limits and taking a closer look at how our perceptions shape what we see and feel. When we do this, we open up space for more empathy, understanding, and flexibility. It's about moving away from rigid "shoulds" and learning to approach life in a way that's more adaptable and open to growth, for us and the people we care about.

The key is to accept that life and relationships are complex. Instead of holding onto unrealistic standards or giving up when things aren't perfect, we can find balance in the middle. This is where the *Gray Area* comes in, a mindset that embraces flexibility and acknowledges the nuances of life. Parenting and relationships do best when approached with humility and curiosity, where we're willing to explore the space between extremes, whether it's right and wrong, success and failure, or certainty and doubt. When we let go of perfectionism and allow imperfection to be part of the process, we create an environment where trust, love, and resilience can thrive.

Stepping into the Gray Area is about finding that sweet spot where real growth happens. It's the space where parents learn to roll with the punches, kids feel free to be themselves, and relationships are built on understanding rather than rigid expectations. This is where we find harmony in the chaos and learn to see the beauty in the imperfect. It's not about getting it right all the time; it's about showing up, staying open, and growing together.

Notes

1. Bertrand Russell, *An Inquiry Into Meaning and Truth* (W W Norton & Co., 1940).
2. Bruce D. Perry, and Oprah Winfrey, *What Happened to You?: Conversations On Trauma, Resilience, and Healing*, 2nd ed. (Flatiron Books, 2021).
3. Jennifer S. Willis, ed., *A Lifetime of Peace: Essential Writings by and About Thich Nhat Hanh* (Da Capo Press, 2003).
4. Joanne K. Rowling, *Harry Potter and the Prisoner of Azkaban* (Bloomsbury Children's Books, 2014).

3

Gray Area

"Happiness is when what you think, what you say, and what you do are in harmony."

—Gandhi

PICTURE THIS: IT's bedtime, and your kid is refusing to brush their teeth. You've got two boxes in front of you—Box A says, "Give in and let them skip brushing for the night," and Box B says, "Stand your ground and prepare for a meltdown." It's easy to believe those are your only choices. What if you added a Box C that says, "Let's brush our teeth together and make it a game," or even a Box D, "Try out that funky new toothpaste that turns your mouth blue"?[i] Suddenly, you've got more options and, we hope, a lot less drama. All it takes is stepping outside the boxes we often confine ourselves to.

---

[i] As a side note, I want to give a massive shout-out to my mother for utilizing Box C on most nights of my childhood; that still sticks in my head today every time I brush my teeth (let me rephrase, on the off chance I remember). She used to sing us the "Twist and Shout" by the Beatles, and when it got to the "ah, ah, ah" part, we used to gargle and spit out our toothpaste. This atmosphere was filled with joy, laughter, and a lot of toothpaste cleanup for my mom, but never a fight, only positivity and successful brushing.

37

As parents, we often fall into this trap, thinking there are only two options in any given situation: either we're nailing this whole parenting thing or we're failing miserably. And when we feel like we're not doing enough, it's easy to spiral into self-doubt. That kind of black-and-white thinking leaves no space for grace, creativity, or self-compassion. Parenting isn't about perfect choices; it's about showing up, learning on the fly, and realizing there's usually more than one right answer, a smorgasbord of options. It's a messy mix of trying your best and simply surviving the day. As I write this, I feel it too—the weight of it all. Some moments I feel like I've got a handle on things. Other times, one tantrum can make me feel like I've completely failed. And I hate to admit it, but there are days I don't have the patience or compassion my kids deserve as little humans fighting their own battles. Life with kids is chaotic and unpredictable. For adults, most daily decisions are fairly binary: pay the bill or don't, respond to the email or ignore it. But with parenting, every choice feels like a mini "choose your own adventure" story, where every option seems like it could go beautifully right or wildly wrong. And unlike the books, there's no flipping back a few pages to undo your choice if it goes sideways.

For example, my three-year-old woke up buzzing with excitement because Grandma was taking him to his favorite place: the land of DINOSAURS! Yes, folks, dinosaurs, the current obsession that has taken over our lives, our bedtime stories, our playroom, and my inability to pronounce "Parasaurolophus" or "Pachycephalosaurus" without embarrassing myself. My son was ready to bolt out the door before breakfast. The problem? The exhibit wasn't open yet. And let me tell you, waiting is not his strong suit. For the next two hours, he repeated the phrase, "It's late!" roughly 372 times. I didn't count, but my nerves felt each one.

In my head, I saw two boxes:

Box A: By the twentieth time, I could lose it. Let the sass fly and yell, "For the love of all things Jurassic, the store isn't open yet! WE HAVE TO WAIT!"

Box B: Muster all the patience I could and be kind and understanding. Acknowledge his excitement and his struggle to wait and gently reassure him that the time would come soon.

But here's what I didn't see until later:

Box C: Ignore it with kindness. Let him feel his feelings, validate it once or twice, and stop trying to explain, fix, or reason with him, because honestly nothing you say will change the outcome, because they don't understand what you are saying.

And you know what? It worked!

When I stopped engaging, something miraculous happened. He wandered into his playroom and got lost in his own little world, where dinosaurs roared. He was jumping off the couch and living his best life. I sat nearby, quietly trying not to get noticed or bothered again, marveling at how quickly he moved on without my intervention. Grandma and the exhibit didn't even cross his mind for the rest of the next 35 minutes.

This was a lightbulb moment for me. As parents, we're so quick to jump into action mode, explaining, soothing, and solving. It's like we're hardwired to be the fix-it people. But sometimes, stepping back and doing *nothing* is the most powerful thing we can do. Who knew that not engaging could be so freeing?

It's not always easy to find humor or grace in these situations. Like the time my son insisted he needed to wear dinosaur pajamas to bed (he has 10 pairs). The problem? They were in the laundry, still crusty from whatever adventure he'd had the day before. Cue full-blown meltdown.

I tried reasoning with him—pointing out the many other perfectly good pajama options, but logic doesn't stand a chance against dino devotion. So I pulled out my go-to move: distraction. I broke into a silly song and rotated through my usual characters (I've got three: Gorilla, Monster, and Chef Flushenflashin). Did it work? Absolutely not. But at least I tried.

See how I ended that paragraph? *At least I tried.* Box C (the Gray Area) is the focus of this chapter. You aren't a failure because the plan didn't work out as you hoped, but at least you tried and *did your best.*

As both a therapist and a dad, I've seen how black-and-white thinking sneaks into relationships, especially in the day-to-day grind. Take something as simple as deciding who's going to handle the next diaper change or bedtime routine. Suddenly, it turns into an unspoken or sometimes loudly spoken competition: Who's done more today? Who did it last?

The mental scoreboard goes up, and before you know it, you're stuck in the loop of "I do everything around here" versus "They're not pulling their weight." It's exhausting, and all too easy for parents to fall into the trap of tallying tasks instead of working as a team.

In 1979, researchers conducted an eye-opening study with thousands of couples, asking each partner to assess how much they contributed to the relationship. The results? Both partners consistently claimed they were doing 120% of the work. Now, I'm no math expert, but even I know that if both of you are doing "everything," someone's numbers aren't adding up. Clearly, no one was sitting around binge-watching TV while the other ran the entire household, but that's how it might have felt to each person. This phenomenon led to the coining of a term called *unconscious claiming.*[1]

Unconscious claiming happens when we instinctively overestimate our own contributions to the shared responsibilities of the home or life while downplaying what others do. Why? Because we vividly remember all the times *we* sacrificed sleep for our sick kids, did carpool, or cleaned up the mess that followed play time with the kids. But we're far less tuned into our partner's efforts, whether it's organizing the bills, folding endless piles of laundry, or doing bedtime. We unconsciously inflate our role while unintentionally minimizing theirs, which can lead to some awkward moments like "You never help with dinner!" as they stand there stirring spaghetti.

This kind of bias might not be intentional, but it can create friction in relationships. Over time, keeping mental scorecards can lead to resentment, frustration, and the dreaded "Who does more?" argument that never ends well. I've been in those arguments myself and have sat with countless couples as they work through the painful, often toxic words that come out during those moments. But recognizing that we're all a little prone to this unconscious claiming is the first step toward more teamwork and fewer passive-aggressive sighs while loading the dishwasher.

Something I teach all my couples is: *you can't quantify quality.* This means to the person doing the actions, that quality is important, whether it's seven things or thirty, it's not about the number but the effort they took. To them, it mattered, and it's hard to convince them otherwise.

Maybe one partner handled seven things that took hours of emotional and mental labor, while the other completed thirty quick tasks in an afternoon. It's not about the numbers and comparing the amount; it's about recognizing and respecting the *quality* of what your partner brings to the table.

Active Tip #1: Just Say Thank You

I utilize this many times in my own life as well as work with clients on this very simple actionable tip: start saying thank you. It has to be for everything and anything. Even if it was planned, even if it was their "job"—say it anyway. In that moment, show them that you see them. Unconscious scorekeeping often stems from feeling unseen or unappreciated. But when we start to notice and express gratitude actively, it shifts our mindset. We stop tallying who did what and start recognizing that we're both working hard to survive the chaos of parenting.

Gratitude is one of the most effective antidotes to anger, annoyance, and resentment. It's hard to truly feel thankful and furious at the same time.

So look for the small things—dishes done, bedtime handled, that mystery object finally removed from the counter—and name it. Appreciate it. You're not just giving thanks; you're training your brain to see your partner again. To recognize their efforts. To move out of "me versus you" and back into "us."

Activity Tip #2: Treasure Hunting

A couple of years ago, I had a wonderful conversation[2] with one of the leading experts in positive psychology (Dr. Sasha Heinz), and she used a terminology called positive hunting. *I loved it—and started using a version of it with my clients and in my own life. I call it* treasure hunting.

The idea is simple but powerful: take a moment to reflect on your day and notice the good, the bad, and everything in between. This isn't about slapping a silver lining on hard things or pretending everything's fine when it's not. It's about making space to see the full picture. Because often, the negative stuff is so loud—so consuming— that we miss the moments of connection, effort, or joy that are also there.

Treasure hunting helps shift the negativity to the edges of your awareness—not to ignore it but to give the positives room to come into focus. It allows your mind and heart to actually register those meaningful moments, instead of being buried under frustration or stress.

Even doing this for just 5–10 minutes during the day or sometime throughout the week can reset your perspective. It won't erase your struggles, but it can offer a much-needed pause. It's a small mental pivot—a way to step back from the spiral of resentment or the tornado of anger, and breathe in a little lightness. There's some goodness in your day. This practice helps you find it.

The Wise Mind

There is a wonderful concept in dialectical behavioral therapy (DBT) called *wise mind*. Just imagine you're standing in the middle of a chaotic morning: the kids are arguing over who gets the last drops of chocolate syrup, your partner is rushing because they have to get to work, and the dog is barking because she wants to go for a walk.

In moments like this, it's easy to react purely from emotion or impulse. I know that struggle personally—living with ADHD and being a parent has stretched every part of my nervous system. That's where DBT has been a game changer.

This is where DBT comes into play, which is basically a fancy term for a practical approach to managing those I'm-about-to-lose-it moments in parenting and life. It helps us find balance in high-stress situations by teaching us to respond with intention instead of reacting on autopilot. At times, parenting can feel like juggling flaming swords while riding a unicycle, but DBT gives us tools to stay grounded.

At the heart of it is the idea that we all have three states of mind: the Emotional Mind, the Rational Mind, and the Wise Mind (that quiet, grounded part of us where reason and emotion work together). When those three are in sync, we make better decisions that reflect both who we are and who we want to be.

Here's how it looks in real life: Your toddler just had a total meltdown because you gave them the *red* cup instead of the sacred *green* one. Your emotional mind is on fire and screaming, "Seriously? After everything I do for you, this is what sets you off?" Meanwhile, your Rational Mind is trying to avoid World War III by swapping cups and moving on. But then there's that quiet voice of inner wisdom, suggesting, *Hey, this might be a good opportunity to teach some patience and flexibility. You don't have to give in every time.*

DBT encourages us to pause and let all parts of ourselves—emotional, rational, and wise—have a voice. Instead of reacting on impulse, it teaches us to slow down: take a breath, check in with how we feel, consider the facts, and make a choice that reflects our values and the bigger picture.

In that "green cup versus red cup" moment, Wise Mind might guide you to calmly explain that the green cup isn't available, while still offering comfort, because even if it's just a cup to you, it's a big deal to them.

One thing I find myself repeating, both to the parents I work with and to myself during those "what on Earth is happening?" moments is this: we're not always going to understand why our kids are upset. We don't have to fully grasp their logic to honor their feelings. Even when their perspective seems puzzling or irrational, what we *can* see is that they're annoyed, upset, and frustrated in that moment. And that's what we need to focus on.

Instead of getting caught up in trying to make sense of their "why," our job is to respond to their emotions and feelings, even when we're scratching our heads in confusion. It's about letting our kids know we're there for them, no matter what. That is what true sympathy is: *I see you have feelings, I care about you and your feelings, so they matter.*

This approach isn't just useful for toddler meltdowns. It's a tool for thriving in all corners of parenting and relationships. Whether it's navigating your teen's eye rolls or trying not to lose it when your partner forgets—again—to put their clothes away, Wise Mind can help you stay grounded.

Here's another example: your partner has left their clothes on the floor for the third time. Emotional Mind wants to explode. Rational Mind is crafting the perfect passive-aggressive comment. But Wise Mind steps in and gently asks, *"Is this really the hill I want to die on?"* You take a breath and realize the frustration is less about the clothes and more about feeling unseen or unappreciated.

From that place of clarity, you might choose to move the clothes for now and later open up an honest conversation about your feelings. The beauty of DBT is that it doesn't ask you to silence your emotions or become some hyper-logical robot who never reacts. Instead, it encourages you to acknowledge and respect your emotions while also considering the facts and your deeper values. This way, you can make decisions that not only solve the immediate problem but also contribute to healthier, more fulfilling relationships with your partner and kids.

So, the next time you're caught in a parenting dilemma, whether it's about dealing with a meltdown, balancing chores, or figuring out how to get some much-needed alone time, try channeling your inner DBT guru. Take a breath, listen to your emotions, weigh the facts, and let your wise mind guide you to a choice that feels right for you and your family. You might just find that with a little practice, making choices from a place of inner wisdom becomes your new parenting superpower.

The Power of Good Enough

Years ago, I read this piece in one of the many Brené Brown books that have blessed our world with compassion, reality, and grace:

"Wholeheartedness: Worthy now. Not if. Not when. We are worthy of love and belonging now. Right this minute. As is. Wholehearted living is about engaging in our lives from a place of worthiness. It means cultivating the courage, compassion, and connection to wake up in the morning and think, no matter what gets done and how much is left undone, I am enough. It's going to bed at night thinking, yes, I am imperfect and vulnerable and sometimes afraid, but that doesn't change the truth that I am also brave and worthy of love and belonging."[3]

Have you ever woken up in the morning with the feeling that today is going to be a massive failure and dumped so much hatred on yourself, before you've even faced the things that the day brings?

Recently, as I mentioned earlier, we went to Disneyland, a place that is considered one of the happiest places on Earth. Before we even went on the trip, about a month or so prior, I was already going through all the issues, failures, and points of triggers that could potentially happen. I was bracing for failure before we even left.

Did some of those things actually happen? Of course.

But did all that mental prepping and rumination change the outcome? Not at all.

All it really did was cast a cloud over the whole experience before it even began. That anxiety bled into how I talked about the trip with my wife, how I prepared for it, and how I showed up during the trip itself. Instead of feeling excitement or possibility, I was stuck in my own fog—unable to see the joy because I was too busy preparing for disappointment.

As parents, we need to learn to accept our limitations, knowing we can't do it all or be perfect all the time. But at the same time, we can choose to live in the present with a sense of positivity and wholeheartedness. As Brené Brown reminds us, *you are worthy of good right now*, regardless of what the outcome may be later.

Don't let the black and white of life put you into a submission of failure and dismay. Instead, step into the possibility of what *could be*, and trust that you have the strength and resilience to handle whatever comes your way. And if you mess up, and you will, you will learn from it and grow to be a better and more well-rounded human.

There's a saying I particularly hate: "What doesn't kill you makes you stronger."[ii]

Why do I hate it you ask?

It sounds powerful, sure—but in practice, it can feel dismissive. Like you're *supposed* to bounce back wiser, tougher, and better just because you survived something hard.

The truth? Sometimes the challenges we face knock us down so hard, we're not sure we can get back up. And often, what doesn't kill you doesn't make you feel stronger at all—it just leaves you hurting.

As someone who's been through tough seasons myself and who's walked alongside many incredible humans facing unthinkable challenges, I've come to believe a better way to put it is this: *What doesn't kill you will test you. It might hurt, it might crush you for a while.* But eventually, if you give yourself the space and support, you can learn from it. You may not come out feeling like a superhero—but you might come out more aware, more grounded, and better equipped to navigate the next storm.

Radical Acceptance Will Set You Free

There is one last piece of practical advice left with this concept of finding the gray and learning a balance of life, and that is acceptance, which for a lot of us is the hardest thing to do.

[ii] Friedrich Nietzsche, but also Kelly Clarkson.

Over COVID, like many, I felt out of control and at a massive loss. But as a therapist I had to learn how to handle my own emotions and feelings, trapped in a small apartment with a baby and working with clients going through the same thing! I felt overwhelmed and in a sick version of *Groundhog Day*, and I was starting to lose where my issues ended and my clients began.

What truly helped me was a tactic called *radical acceptance*, which can be broken down into three easy steps:

(1) This Happened
(2) I Feel
(3) Now What

This Happened: This is the ability to name what is going on in your life and giving it a space to breathe and live outside of all the noise of feelings, for example:

- "I am a parent whose baby can't sleep for more than three to four hours."
- "I am not getting much sleep."
- "My wife and I keep fighting and we haven't had sex in more than two months."
- "I'm struggling as a father."
- "Work has been taking me away from kid time."
- "I just screamed at my kids, and I don't know why."

The goal here is to name what's happening, without judgment or interpretation. Just state the facts.

I Feel: This is where things get energized.

- "I feel overwhelmed and scared for how the next few months will go and I can't see the light with all the anger and frustration I feel."
- "I feel sad that my partner and I might get divorced. What's going to happen to the baby?"
- "I feel alone as a dad. I'm not sure if I'm cut out for this."

- "I feel like I am hurting my kids by not being around and am filled with so much guilt that I can't look at myself in the morning."
- "I feel like such a failure as a parent because I made my kid cry. All he did was ask for help. What is wrong with me?"

This is letting our emotions flow and be felt without holding back or hiding from the truth of what we feel. Again, *no judgment*.

Now What: This is where we realize we can't change what has happened or sometimes what is currently happening, but we are going to accept the reality of now and figure out how we can best live within the truth of today. It doesn't always feel sexy or can be uncomfortable at times, but for us to get through life, it's the only way to live.

- "I can't make my baby sleep through the night, but I *can* take a 20-minute nap when someone offers to help or asks for help even when it's hard."
- "My wife and I aren't connecting right now, but tonight I'll put my phone down and ask her one question about her day, and just listen."
- "I can't undo the yelling, but I *can* apologize to my kid, take a breath, and remind myself that I'm still a good parent who's learning."
- "Work is demanding, but I can set a timer for 10 minutes tonight to play with my kid fully present, even if it's just rolling cars or reading the same book for the hundredth time."
- "I'm feeling distant from my partner, but I can leave a sticky note on the fridge that says, 'I know we're both tired. I still love you.'"
- "I'm struggling as a father, but I can talk to a friend, therapist, or another dad and remind myself that I don't have to carry this alone."
- "I feel overwhelmed, but I *can* take three deep breaths before walking into the next room and that counts as a win today."

Back to the COVID example, here is the breakdown I did:

This Happened/This Is: COVID is here, and I have no idea how to handle life right now.

I Feel: I feel trapped, overwhelmed, and unsure about how our life is going to be in the next week, month, or years, and honestly, I am a bit scared of what world I am raising my kids in. I'm at a loss.

Now What: I asked myself what I needed to do to feel as comfortable as I could with my feelings and realities. I spoke honestly with my clients about how they were feeling and shared some of my truths about the situation. I had a real conversation with my wife about how to make the life we were in a bit less stifling (we picked up and moved into my in-law's house in Los Angeles for five months to get out of our apartment, get some needed help, and be outdoors a bit more).

The key to acceptance isn't necessarily liking what you accept but dealing with it in a smarter, better, and more productive way than before.

I'll give you another example that has and will probably continue to impact my life, relationship, and parenting: I have Crohn's disease. I was diagnosed when I was 18 and went through some really tough times over the years due to it.

It took me a very long time to accept the reality of my chronic illness and the ways it would impact my life, whether I liked it or not. There have been and continue to be changes I need to make in my life to ensure I stay healthy and stable.

When my wife and I first started dating and in the early years of our marriage, plans were canceled, and life was put on hold due to my being very sick, in the hospital, or just in the bathroom.

Acceptance helped me free myself from the burden of guilt that I carried. I was able to look at myself without judgment because I wasn't doing anything wrong; I just had Crohn's.

The same thing goes for parenting and our kids. Your kid is who they are today, behaving in whatever manner they may be. Screaming or getting so dysregulated won't change them or the fact that they are three and can't handle a long car ride. As adults, we need to take a moment for radical acceptance: *This is, I Feel, Now What.*

Journey to Balanced Thinking

The thing about black-and-white thinking is that it's comfortable; it helps make things easier to do on the fly when life is so stressful. Especially in the middle of parenting chaos, it's so tempting to simplify everything into "good" or "bad," just to keep yourself sane. It's tempting to think, "This is right, that's wrong." End of story. When your toddler is screaming, "Are we there yet"? Every 10–15 seconds on a 5-hour car drive, and it's hard to find space for nuance in those moments.

It gives us a sense of certainty in a world that's anything but certain. Black-and-white thinking offers certainty, but real life happens in the gray. And that's where the magic is, where growth, connection, and possibility live.

Black-and-white thinking also has a sneaky way of creeping into how we view ourselves as parents. On a rough day, it's easy to jump to "I'm a terrible parent because I lost my cool" or "I'm the best parent ever because I made homemade cookies."

I recently had to practice finding the gray area when one of my children cried as I got them out of bed. "You're not Mommy. I don't like you, Daddy." They went on to cry for 20–30 minutes straight that mommy is working and this stranger (me) isn't good enough. They wanted a snack or help with something, and I was right there to help, but I got yelled at. "No, I want Mommy to get it," and she wasn't even in the room.

It's easy to fall into a deep pain of failure and not know what you're doing wrong. I've had that thought more times than I care to admit this month. But parenting isn't an all-or-nothing game.

Some days you're the silly and amazing hero, and other days you're the parent who just needs a moment to breathe before facing the next challenge. Both are okay, and both are part of the journey.

Life and parenting rarely fit into those tidy categories. It's more like a giant cluttered middle. Think about those moments when you're convinced you're either the world's best parent or totally screwing it up. One minute, you're channeling Bluey's dad, having all the patience in the world, and the best games to entertain your kids for hours. Next, you're overwhelmed and feeling guilty because you snapped at your kid for saying your name for the thirtieth time in three seconds.

Take screen time, for example. How easy is it to fall into the trap of "It's either all screens, all day, or we're going full old-school mode—outdoors, playing with rocks and dirt"? But most of us live somewhere in between. Maybe your kids get a little Disney or Nickelodeon while you get five minutes of hot coffee and silence. That's balance, right? And it works.

What I've learned is that parenting is more like abstract art than a black-and-white photograph. You know, the kind of painting where some people see brilliance and others are like, "Is this upside down?" or "My 2-year-old can make that." That's family life. It's colorful, unpredictable, sometimes chaotic and, yeah, kind of beautiful.

When we stop trying to squeeze everything into two tiny boxes, we open ourselves up to all sorts of possibilities. We can be more flexible, more forgiving of ourselves and others, and a lot more creative in finding solutions that work for everyone.

When we let go of the all-or-nothing mindset, a weight lifts. Suddenly, your partner isn't the villain who loaded the dishwasher *wrong* or is taking a moment to breathe by scrolling their phone and doesn't deserve the death stare from across the room; they're just another tired human doing their best, like you. Maybe instead of throwing them shade, you hand out a high-five, a longer hug and a tushy squeeze.

So, the next time you catch yourself stuck in black-and-white thinking, remember that there's a whole spectrum of grays out there. Maybe it's not about choosing between two extremes but about finding a balance somewhere in the middle, or even outside the box altogether. Parenting isn't about getting it right all the time; it's about navigating the in-betweens, finding joy in the unexpected, and knowing that it's okay to color outside the lines.

And while we're exploring balance, it's essential to address self-care. Black-and-white thinking often pushes it to the bottom of our priority list, as if it's optional or indulgent. Just like the well-known advice to put on your own oxygen mask before helping others, the principle holds: you can't pour from an empty cup. When you're depleted, the stress and chaos of daily life spill over more easily. Prioritizing your well-being isn't selfish; it's foundational to showing up as the parent and partner you want to be.

Notes

1. Ross and Sicoly (1979), Kruger and Savitsky (2009), Schroeder (2017).
2. *The Dude Therapist*. "Let's Get Unstuck and Create a Life of Meaning." *The Dude Therapist*, hosted by Eli Weinstein, guest Dr. Sasha Heinz, 21 Aug. 2022.
3. Brené Brown, *The Gifts of Imperfection: Let Go of Who You Think You're Supposed to Be and Embrace Who You Are* (Hazelden, 2010).

4

Oxygen Tank

"To love oneself is the beginning of a lifelong romance."

—Oscar Wilde

YOU'RE FLYING IN for the holidays with your kids to see your parents. You walk in the door after a long five-hour flight and several diaper and outfit changes. You're genuinely looking forward to reconnecting with your parents, but what happens? They run to greet your child, while you stand there with your three bags, two suitcases, and a baby carrier. Now, I'll admit, as a parent, seeing your child have a village of people love on your kids is truly the best thing ever. However, it can sometimes lead to a common feeling as parents, that in this new chapter of our lives, we are no longer the top priority.

So much of our time has and continues to be all about our kids, from the second we wake up to even while we sleep. Our priorities of life have changed, our rhythm of life has changed, and the needs of the people around us have changed. But for some reason, we stop adjusting with that life, getting stuck in a continuous loop of putting ourselves far down the list of things that matter.

We don't ask parents how they truly are doing because they magically fall away once the kids come into play. Let me ask you something often overlooked: how are you, really?

53

Along the way, it's easy to fall into the trap of putting your kids' needs ahead of your own, because let's face it, who has time for a bubble bath when there's a toddler trying to get your attention, screaming about who knows what, and not going to bed when they should be. But constantly sacrificing your well-being for the sake of your little ones isn't just unsustainable, it's a recipe for disaster. I see it time and time again with my clients and myself, thinking they are being the best parents to be all in on their kids, no matter when and no matter how, without seeing how it's draining them.

Let this sink in: *you matter so much!*

Without you being at your best, or even just taking care of your basic needs and beyond, you are not just doing a disservice to yourself but also to the world around you.

Enter the Oxygen Mask Principle, aka the best piece of parenting advice no one tells you about until you're already knee-deep in chaos, diapers, and sleepless nights. Now we have all heard it on airplanes during the safety instructions: "Put on your own oxygen mask before assisting others." It's a solid metaphor for parenting, too. If you're running on fumes, you won't have the energy or patience to be the parent or partner you want to be. So, before you dive into solving everyone else's problems, make sure you've got your air supply sorted.

We all have a tank that gets drained differently depending on lack of sleep, hunger, stress, or just the weight of everyday life. The key is being aware of where your tank is at and how that impacts your interactions. I'm not saying you need to be at 100% all the time—that's not realistic. But you do need to be at a level that allows you to function in a way that's healthy for you and helpful for the people around you.

Over the years, both in my practice and in my own marriage, I've heard people say that parenting should be 50/50. And honestly? I disagree. Parenting isn't a fixed split—it's a fluid give-and-take. Some days, you're running on half a tank and giving your all with that half is still giving 100%. What matters is showing up with what you *can* give.

Tip #1: Tank Check-In

In our cars, we have dashboard lights that let us know if we need more gas, if our tires need more air, or if our engine needs a checkup. When it comes to be a human, we don't have any lights that shine on our foreheads to let others know what we need. Often, it comes through with being snippy, isolating, or anxious. Many of us have a hard time verbalizing that we aren't doing okay today.

The action is to just say either "engine light" or "my tank is low." All this does is signal to the people who we've let into this terminology, whether it be our spouse, kids, friends, or parents. This means I need a break, a refill, or to step away for a bit. It's a way to check in with yourself and take the time you need.

Additionally, if someone in your life is aware of your tendencies and baseline and feels you are off or struggling (for whatever reason and there doesn't need to be an explanation), they can ask, "How is your tank?"

This should not become a game for whose tank is lower or who needs a break more. This is someone in the relationship being extremely honest and vulnerable with how they are doing, and they deserve the utmost respect at that crucial relationship trust moment. It may be that you are both extremely low due to life and everything that goes along with it and you need to push through on an empty tank, but you always have each other's back through the lows of the tank.

Now, I know what you're thinking: "Self-care? Who has time for that?" Trust me, I get it. Between the school runs, food shopping, work, making dinner, tantrums, walking the dog, and the never-ending pile of laundry and toys to clean up, self-care can feel like a distant dream.

Self-care isn't about finding time; it's about making time. It's about recognizing that taking care of yourself isn't selfish; it's essential. After all, you wouldn't expect a car to get anywhere on an empty tank, so why do you expect the same from yourself?

We are not going to talk about unrealistic self-care; we are going to deal with the internal self-care that all humans deserve for their well-being and, let's be honest, sanity throughout the struggles of life.

When we hear the phrase *self-care*, our minds often jump to luxurious escapes: spa days, weekend getaways, or serene retreats. And while those moments are wonderful (and ideally on your calendar at some point), that's not the daily reality for most parents. For us, self-care often looks far more modest: five quiet minutes with a cup of coffee, a quick walk around the block, or simply sitting alone in the bathroom, doing absolutely nothing for a moment, just breathing, scrolling, or enjoying a rare bit of silence. These small, intentional pauses are not frivolous. They're powerful. And they're necessary. Self-care doesn't have to be grand to be meaningful; it just has to exist.

Here's the magic of self-care: it doesn't benefit just you. When you take care of yourself, you're also taking care of your relationships. Think about it: when you're feeling good, you're more patient, more present, and much less likely to snap at your partner for leaving dirty socks on the floor. By investing in yourself, you're also investing in the people you love. Your kids get a happier, more relaxed parent, and your partner gets someone who's not just surviving, but enjoying life.

When I don't journal, listen to my music, or move my body in some way, I'm not that pleasant to be around. And the worst part is, I don't even notice it sometimes. I turn into a bit of an ogre, stomping around my house and destroying the parts of my life that matter most, which are my wife and kids. I push myself aside to see one more client, do that podcast recording, or edit a social media post.

The "just one more thing" mindset is often what sabotages my self-care. It's this inner monologue of not being enough, doing enough, or doing more compared to _____ (fill in whoever I am admiring or following on social media that day).

While writing this amazing book, I have tried to take 10–15 minutes of self-care a day, which isn't much, but it's a non-negotiable for my sanity. It's a challenge to look at my day and prioritize myself without feeling a dooming sense of guilt and questioning if I even earned this break.

Isn't that wild? We question ourselves if we earned the 10–15 minutes of a longer shower, reading, or just peace and quiet! You absolutely deserve that time and you don't need to earn it. You deserve it simply because you're human and navigating life, stress, responsibilities…and, on top of that, keeping little humans alive while trying to hold everything together.

So let me be clear: breaks aren't bonuses. They're basic survival. Take them. No guilt, no debate, no justification needed.

In the constant demands of parenting and relationships, it's easy to put yourself at the very bottom of the list. You tell yourself there's no time, that your kids or your partner need you more, that self-care can wait. But what if taking care of yourself is the very thing that allows you to show up better for your family, for your marriage, and for the life you're building together?

So, as you navigate the ups and downs of parenting, remember to put on your oxygen mask first. It's not just about surviving; it's about thriving. When you take time to refuel, even in small ways, your relationships become stronger, more connected, and more fulfilling. In the end, a little self-care can go a long way in keeping the whole family running smoothly.

In her book *Start Where You Are*, Buddhist teacher Pema Chödrön makes an insightful observation: "What you do for yourself, you're doing for others, and what you do for others, you're doing for yourself."[1] It's a reminder that self-care is not a solo act; it's a ripple. When you treat yourself with kindness, patience, and compassion, those qualities inevitably flow into your relationships. The care you give yourself becomes the foundation for the care you give your family.

Think about those days when you're running on fumes, trying to give your kids everything they need while balancing the weight of the world. What happens? You're shorter with them, less present, and less able to respond with the love and patience you want to give. The same thing happens in your marriage. Exhaustion makes you snap at small things, avoid deeper conversations, or withdraw because there's just nothing left in the tank. Self-care isn't just about feeling better; it's about having the capacity to show up as the best version of yourself for the people you love.

Tending to your own needs is a quiet way of saying, "I'm worth it." It's about tuning in to your needs and creating a sense of balance. That might be carving out 30 minutes to exercise, saying "no" to one more obligation, or simply allowing yourself to sit down and rest without guilt. These small acts of self-respect send a powerful message to your family: *I matter, and my well-being matters.* Parenting isn't just about what we say; it's about what we model. When you make time to care for yourself, you're showing your children what it looks like to prioritize mental, emotional, and physical health. They're watching you. You're showing them how to handle stress, honor their needs, and approach life with compassion, not just for others but for themselves too.

The same is true in marriage. When you and your partner each take responsibility for your individual well-being, it strengthens the bond between you. You bring more energy, patience, and openness to the relationship. You listen better, support each other more fully, and are less likely to build resentment. When one person feels constantly depleted, the balance of the relationship shifts, creating tension or distance. But when you both commit to self-care, it becomes a shared value— something that benefits not just the individual but the partnership.

Tip #2: Mound Visit

This might seem like a simple tip to implement in your relationship, and many of the couples I've worked with are shocked and amazed by how much of a difference it can make.

If you have ever watched baseball, there is something called a mound visit. *It's when a teammate, coach, or usually the catcher walks up to the pitcher during a tough moment. They have a quick check-in to see how the pitcher is really doing. Then they talk through a game plan for what's coming next.*

> *If you see your partner isn't at their baseline, just pull them aside and ask two simple questions:*
>
> (1) *How are you doing?*
> (2) *How can I help you get back to your baseline?*
>
> *This shows you see them for their struggles and gives them the opening to know you are willing to help when they ask. It creates an environment of love and comfort and a plan of action.*

There's also an emotional spillover that happens when you care for yourself. You become more centered, more grounded, and more capable of showing up with genuine love. When you take time to recharge, you're able to handle the inevitable chaos of family life with greater ease. The tantrums, the messes, the disagreements, they don't feel as overwhelming when you're not running on empty. Your family feels the difference in your energy and presence, even if they don't fully understand why.

There was a rough patch I was having for a couple of weeks, and I wasn't my usual cheery, silly self. I was in my head about many different things in life. When I started tuning into my needs and taking care of myself, my wife looked at me and said, "There you are!" I was back to myself, which in turn made it a better zone for everyone else in the home.

And let's not forget how much your marriage benefits when you're both in a healthier space. Intimacy thrives when you're not burdened by constant fatigue or resentment. A little self-care can reignite connection and bring more joy into your partnership. It might mean having the energy to laugh together at the end of the day, being more patient in the face of challenges, or simply having the capacity to hold space for each other's emotions without feeling stretched too thin.

When you care for yourself, you're not just filling your own cup. You're filling the cups of everyone around you. You're creating a healthier, happier family dynamic, where love, respect, and compassion flow freely. And in doing so, you're not just taking care of yourself, you're taking care of the people who mean the most to you.

Tip #3: Self-Care Card

We don't often know when we need help to get us out of a funky headspace or a rough patch. I encourage you to sit down with a 3 × 5 card and jot down all the things that truly fill your cup. Some examples for me:

- *A nice cup of tea*
- *Reading*
- *Playing a board game with my wife*
- *Taking a walk with my dog*
- *Gym/sauna*
- *Snuggling with my kids/wife*

These are just a few. Don't hold back when making your list. List all the big and small things that can lift you up and fill your tank. Now take three different color highlighters/markers:

(1) Green/blue: Easy effort/quick refill
(2) Yellow/orange: Middle effort/medium refill
(3) Red: Most effort/fills your tank to the fullest

If you need to rewrite on a new card, go for it. Make it yours!
Once you are done with the system, share it with your spouse and talk it through so they are in the know. When you say you need a green, yellow, or red right now, they know what you are talking about. Next, put it somewhere accessible like your bedside table, office, or fridge so you can reference it when things get rough.
Let this be your self-care cheat sheet.

Feed the Beast

We all fall into habits or strategies that once worked well and now simply run on autopilot. In parenting, these patterns can quietly shift from helpful routines to unconscious defaults.

The term is called *feeding the beast*; this comes from a story in the book *Creativity, Inc.* about Pixar's early days. After the massive success of *Toy Story*, the studio rushed into a sequel, assuming that slapping the same title on a new story would automatically re-create the magic. But it didn't. The film lacked heart, clarity, and direction. Midway through production, they realized they were no longer creating something meaningful; they were just trying to satisfy demand. That's feeding the beast: relying on what's familiar, what's easy, what once worked, without stopping to ask if it still serves us.

And the beast is always hungry.

It demands content, results, and output. Feeding the beast feels like the easy choice, the path of least resistance. The problem is that it doesn't always lead to success. And it rarely leads to joy.

As parents, we often fall back on the tactics or routines that once helped us survive a tough moment—a special story, a silly voice, a promise of extra snuggles. And because it worked, we label it: "This works." So we repeat it. Again and again. Over time, we slip into autopilot: copy, paste, repeat. It feels efficient. Maybe even safe.

But what worked yesterday might not be what your child or you need today.

When we stop reflecting and start reacting out of habit, we're not being intentional; we're feeding the beast. That beast is burnout, disconnection, and emotional detachment. It's the part of parenting where we do what's familiar, not necessarily what's best.

Think about it: are there routines or reactions you've put on repeat just because they once got you through a tough night or phase? Maybe it's how you handle tantrums, rely on bribes, or check out emotionally when you're drained. Autopilot might feel like a shortcut, but over time, it can wear you down and create distance— from your kids, your partner, and even yourself.

When you recognize the beast in your own parenting—the relentless push to do more, repeat what worked, or perform perfection—it's a cue to pause. Ask yourself: *Is this still working? Is this the version of myself I want to bring to my family today?*

We don't defeat the beast by doing more. We reset by doing differently intentionally, consciously, and with care for ourselves and those we love.

This is where self-care becomes essential. When you're constantly running on empty, feeding the beast becomes the default. It's easier to copy and paste what you've always done than to pause, reflect, and ask yourself: "What's actually needed here?" Self-care gives you the space and energy to respond with intention, not just habit. It helps you show up as the A-team version of yourself, not the B-team running on fumes.

And no, self-care isn't always easy. When you're juggling parenting, relationships, and everything else, it can feel impossible. But it starts with small moments of awareness—recognizing when you're stuck in the loop, giving yourself permission to step back, and asking, "Is this still working?" or "Is this what we need right now?" Sometimes, even five quiet minutes, a deep breath, or a slight shift in routine can help disrupt the cycle.

Self-care isn't about luxury; It's how we reclaim our energy and reconnect with the clarity and compassion we need to lead our families with heart.

The team at Pixar once scrapped an entire movie, losing millions of dollars, just to get the story right. That's a steep price. As parents, the cost isn't money; it's time, energy, and connection. Feeding the beast might get us through a moment, but intentionality helps us build something lasting and meaningful.

It starts with a simple pause: "Is this what's best for my child? For my family? For me?" Sometimes the answer is no, and that's okay. Growth happens in those moments of reflection and course correction.

Parenting isn't about perfection. It's about showing up with presence, honesty, and love. So, let's stop feeding the beast out of habit. Let's give ourselves permission to reset, to care for ourselves, and to rewrite the story, even if it takes a little longer, even if it's a little harder.

Because when we show up as the A-team version of ourselves, *that's* when the real magic happens.

The Power of Ish

Recently, I was reading a wonderful kids' book with my daughter called *Ish* by Peter Reynolds. My daughter has been struggling with wanting her art to be perfect and getting so frustrated when things aren't just right. So, this book seemed like the right fit and perfect story to share with her. The deeper message was a little over her head, but it hit me straight in the heart.

The story is about Ramon, a young boy who loves to draw. For him, creating art is pure joy. It's fun, carefree, and imaginative. But that joy vanishes when his older brother makes a thoughtless comment, laughing at a drawing Ramon had been proud of. Suddenly, doubt creeps in. What once felt playful and fulfilling now feels stressful and frustrating. Ramon becomes obsessed with making his drawings look perfect and, in the process, loses the love he once had for creating.

Just when Ramon is ready to give up, his younger sister, Marisol, steps in and changes everything. She has been quietly saving his discarded drawings, treasuring them for what they are: "ish." A vase doesn't need to look exactly like a vase to be "vase-ish," and for Marisol, that's more than enough. Her gentle encouragement helps Ramon see his art in a whole new way. He realizes that there is beauty in imperfection and that art doesn't need to be flawless to be meaningful.

Reading this to my daughter, I found myself tearing up. Though the book wasn't about parenting, I felt so deeply seen. There is so much pressure to be the best parent and to have it all together and live within the "lines" of what we think good parenting should look like. But I've never been great at staying in the lines. I've always been more about doing my best, appreciating the journey, and finding joy in the messy process.

We feel like we shouldn't get upset at our kids, frustrated at the hardship of parenting, or complain because we are "blessed" to have children. We feel we need to have an amazing job, have the house in order, dinner on the table, and the best games and activities for our kids to be engaged.

Why is it so hard to extend that same grace to myself as a parent or as a partner? Why do I find it so difficult to embrace an "ish" mentality when it comes to my relationships? Dan Harris describes this beautifully, calling it the "ish" moment:

"Make the present moment your friend rather than your enemy because many people live habitually as if the present moment were an obstacle that they need to overcome to get to the next moment. And imagine living your whole life like that, where this moment is never quite right, not good enough because you need to get to the next one. That is continuous stress."[2]

This story hit me hard because I see myself in it. I catch myself constantly rushing toward the next moment, trying to get everything just right, and still feeling like I'm falling short no matter how hard I try. That chase for perfection pulls me out of the present. It consumes my thoughts, tightens my body, and blinds me to the "ish" moments that make life beautiful.

Growing up, my dad used to joke that kids always want to play with the box the amazing toy came in. We spend so much time trying to find the perfect gift, the perfect plan, the perfect experience, but in the end, our kids will find joy in their own way. We're not in control of how they choose to play, laugh, or enjoy life. And maybe that's the point. Our job isn't to script the perfect moments; it's to make space for the *imperfectly wonderful* ones.

We as parents have to be able to step back and let things happen with some "ish" mentality. We do the best we can and see how things go. If our kids are happy, fed, and alive, we are killing it as parents that day. Pat yourself on the back, give you and your partner a huge high five, and hug, and that's more than enough. That's a win.

What if we gave ourselves permission to be "ish" parents? To color outside the lines, make mistakes (and own up to them), and recognize that a microwave meal, takeout, your kids playing with the box the toy came in, or just running around like silly ghosts might be exactly what the day calls for. Someone just told me that they had all these plans for their kid's birthday party, putting in hours of research for the best things to do in the area, planning a theme, coming up with the menu, and making a birthday cake. She finally spoke with her son and asked him what he wanted to do. He said, "I want to go to the park and run around with friends." So that's what they did. That is an "ish" moment of parenting.

The stress of trying to be a perfect parent can weigh us down. But when we let go of perfection and focus on just being, we create space for joy, connection, and real love.

The Art of Compassion

Many of us have likely read the story of the two wolves. It shares a powerful lesson that a grandmother is teaching her grandson.

> "A fight is going on inside me," he said to the boy. "It is a terrible fight, and it is between two wolves. One is evil—he is anger, envy, sorrow, regret, greed, arrogance, self-pity, guilt, resentment, inferiority, lies, false pride, superiority, and ego. The other is good—he is joy, peace, love, hope, serenity, humility, kindness, benevolence, empathy, generosity, truth, compassion, and faith. The same fight is going on inside you—and inside every other person, too." The grandson thought about it for a minute and then asked his grandfather, "Which wolf will win?" The old Cherokee simply replied, "The one you feed."

One of the hardest parts about self-care is the internal narrative we continue to feed ourselves, no matter how hard we work or do great things.

When I was listening to this mother who was in my office more than seven years ago, I was shaken by the constant attack on herself and how she felt worthless, despite all she does for her family:

Sophia: *Eli, I do so much for my kids; I give them love, show up when they get hurt, cook their favorite meals, and take them to school, extracurriculars, and appointments. But there is this inner voice that keeps eating at me telling me I can do more for them. What am I missing out on? What am I doing wrong?*

She listed all the positives but focused only on what was lacking. I have heard this so often from parents over the years and have taught them myself. We become the first target of our criticism and have no grace during the journey and or acknowledgment for the daily work and efforts to create a life for our kids and ourselves.

The inner critic is very strong. Many of us have intense gremlins that are constantly hating on us and feeding the negative voice, especially when we are doing everything right and things are good. They laugh and point a finger at all the "mistakes," missed opportunities, and bumps we go through during the day.

I remember a couple of years ago when my baby was crying uncontrollably. I burped her, fed her, rocked her, sang to her—tried everything I could to calm her down. But she kept crying. And the first thing I did? I turned on myself. "I must be the worst parent. I can't even soothe my own baby." Why is it so hard to truly love ourselves and see the greatness in ourselves for all the hard work we are doing?

Lately, my kids have been more attached to their mother, which I genuinely love and find so sweet. But in the middle of the night, when you stumble out of a deep sleep to comfort a crying child and the first thing you hear is "Get out, I want Mommy!"—it cuts deep.

It's not about jealousy. It's about feeling invisible. Unwanted. And some days, that ache adds up fast. Six times before lunch? Been there.

I remember a friend years ago, in the early trenches of parenting, completely overwhelmed by feelings of inadequacy. He looked at me and said, "I don't think I'm doing enough."

So I asked him three simple questions:

(1) Is your kid alive?
(2) Are they fed?
(3) Are they healthy and happy?

If you can answer *yes* to those basic, vital questions, you're already doing something incredible. And that truth? You can hold onto it when the doubts creep in. Because sometimes, surviving the day *is* the win. And that's more than enough.

Tip #4: See the Light

You've likely felt stuck in self-doubt, questioning your worth as a parent or partner. It's that dark space where nothing feels like enough and everything feels like too much. When those thoughts creep in, try this simple, three-step practice to shift into a more grounded, positive mindset:

Step 1: Get comfortable. Close your eyes. Take a deep breath in, and slowly blow it out like you're blowing out a candle. Let your shoulders drop.

Step 2: Write down or speak aloud the negative thoughts swirling in your mind—those inner gremlins that say you're failing or falling short. Get them out. Name them.

Step 3: Now, name three things you did well today. They don't have to be huge. Maybe your kid made it to school with a jacket, lunch, and a water bottle. Maybe you kept your cool during a meltdown. Maybe you planned something fun for the weekend. Whatever it is, name it.

Hold onto that feeling, that reminder that you are doing enough. You are enough. These small wins are proof of your effort, your care, and your strength. Let that be the voice you carry forward.

The great Dr. Seuss said, "Today you are you! That is truer than true! There is no one alive who is you-er than you! Shout loud, 'I am lucky to be what I am!'"[3] As a dad who's been in the thick of it, that line is something I carry with me when having one of those hard days. Some days, just making it to bedtime feels like a win. You're tired, overwhelmed, maybe even falling apart a little but you're still here. And that counts.

That's what self-care really is. *It's not fluff; it's the fuel.* It's allowing yourself to be human, to have limits, and to stop beating yourself up when things don't go perfectly. Because when it's 3 a.m. and the baby won't sleep, what you need most isn't perfection, it's compassion. The kind you give to others but often forget to give to yourself.

So take a deep breath, let go of the pressure to do it all, and know that showing up is enough. Now let's dive into *Chaos O'clock,* where sleep dies, survival begins, and grace becomes your most powerful relationship tool.

Notes

1. Pema Chödrön, *Start Where You Are: A Guide to Compassionate Living* (Shambhala, 1994). http://ci.nii.ac.jp/ncid/BA61396758.
2. Dan Harris, *10% Happier: How I Tamed the Voice in My Head, Reduced Stress Without Losing My Edge, and Found Self-Help That Actually Works - A True Story* (Dey Street Books, 2014).
3. Dr. Seuss, *Happy Birthday to You!* (Random House, 1987).

5

Chaos O'Clock: Where Sleep Dies and Survival Begins

"Christ, three A.M.! ... Sleep is a patch of death, but three in the morn,
full wide-eyed staring, is living death!"

—Ray Bradbury

MY SON MAX was born in February 2022, and our daughter was around three years old. I felt prepared. I knew what to expect; I was now a "seasoned" parent and was confident we could handle it all again. I had no idea just how much this second round would test us. Little did we know that this was going to be the biggest test of our sanity. Our first go around tested our communication and relationship, but our son pushed everything to the next level.

From the moment we heard "Congratulations, it's a boy," the sleep vanished. For the first year, we barely got any rest. Max had tongue, cheek, and lip ties that made feeding difficult—causing gas, swallowing issues, and endless nighttime crying. His cries didn't just echo through the walls—they stirred up frustration, anger, and self-doubt. They broke us down.

For the first 15 weeks of his life, we took turns sleeping in shifts. He could sleep only on our chests, so we propped ourselves up at just the right angle, terrified to move an inch. If we shifted even slightly, he'd wake up screaming, and the whole night would spiral into chaos again. It was exhausting, relentless, and demoralizing.

That period was one of the hardest times of my life. I could barely think straight, let alone show up as a dad to our 3-year-old, a therapist to my clients, or a loving husband to my wife, who had just undergone a C-section and was surviving the same storm.

I don't think we've ever cried so much or felt so completely drained by parenting. What made it harder was the shock. We thought we knew what we were doing. Our daughter had slept four to five hours at a stretch as a newborn. She didn't nap well, but nighttime was manageable. We naïvely believed all babies would be similar. They're not.

That chapter of our life taught me a hard and humbling truth: every child brings their own challenges, joys, and unknowns. I just wasn't prepared for how far I'd be pushed. Max tested our limits, and while we made it through, we came out the other side bruised, broken, and forever changed.

One of the biggest challenges of sleep deprivation is the toll it has on your relationship. When you're both exhausted, it's easy for tempers to flare and for small annoyances to turn into big arguments. You might find yourselves bickering over who got more sleep (as if you're keeping a tally) or who's more tired. Surprise, you both are! The key here is to cut each other some slack. You're both in survival mode, and it's okay if things aren't running smoothly. Remember, you're on the same team, so instead of keeping score, focus on supporting each other through this rough patch.

Now, I can't believe I'm admitting this, but there was one family meal where I completely broke down. I was crying, yelling, and if I'm being honest, throwing a full-on adult tantrum about our son. I resented him. Not because of who he was, but because of what we were going through. I couldn't access the joy of having a newborn; it was buried beneath layers of exhaustion, fear, and pure survival. I knew I loved him, but all I could feel in that moment was trapped. I couldn't see past the suffering.

There was something else going on during those sleepless nights, something I hadn't anticipated. It was more than just the physical exhaustion; it was a pure, raw fear of what the night would bring. Every evening, as the sun started to set, I'd feel this growing sense of dread and worry. It was almost like I was a kid again, afraid of the dark, only this time, it wasn't monsters under the bed, but the newborn in my arms!

That anxiety weighed on me in ways I'd never experienced before, even with our oldest where I had panic attacks over being a parent. This felt so different. Every night felt like walking into a war zone without knowing where the ambush was coming from. That unpredictability lodged itself deep in my body: tight shoulders, clenched jaw, a permanent knot in my stomach. I was bracing for impact before the night even began, like gearing up for a marathon I hadn't trained for. And that fear didn't stay contained to the night. It followed me into the day. The "what ifs" haunted everything; what if he doesn't nap, what if I snap, what if we just can't do this anymore? It clouded my interactions with my wife, my kids, and my clients. I was operating from a place of constant fight-or-flight, trying to stay afloat in a sea of dysregulation.

Fear and anxiety have a sneaky way of creeping into parenthood. It's not just the sleepless nights that get to you, but also the anticipation of what *could* happen, the fear of the unknown. That anticipation, that dread, can be just as exhausting as the sleep loss itself. But what I've come to realize is this: it's okay to admit when you're struggling, even if the fear feels irrational. Even if no one else seems to be falling apart the way you are. Fear is a natural part of parenting. It doesn't make you weak, it makes you human. And acknowledging it is the first step to finding some peace. We start to loosen our grip. We breathe a little deeper. We remember that we're not alone in this.

Sleep deprivation is brutal. It chips away at your patience, your identity, your connection. But it's also a rite of passage that every parent goes through. It's okay to struggle, to feel overwhelmed, and to count down the minutes until you can crawl back into bed.

And in the midst of the chaos, it's okay to find little moments of joy; to laugh at how absurd it all is, to count down the minutes until bedtime, to cry in the kitchen if you need to. You're doing an amazing job, even if it doesn't feel like it.

So the question is: how do we survive those sleepless nights without losing ourselves or each other in the process? How do we show up with a little more grace, a little more kindness, and just enough energy to stay connected through the fog?

This Town Is Big Enough for the Both of You

Imagine you have had a terrible night with your child. You feel like a zombie, and you look to your partner and say, "Honey, I am SOO tired." A lot of people would embrace that with love, a hug, or some measure of kindness, but your partner is also tired. All they hear is "I had a worse night than you, and I am more tired than you," and the frustrations build.

Something I work on with many of my clients and with myself is this: two truths can exist at the same time. Your experience doesn't cancel out your partner's. There's enough space for both of your suffering to matter. Just because you're hurting doesn't mean they're not. And just because they're struggling doesn't mean your pain disappears.

When both of you are exhausted, it's tempting to compete for whose pain is bigger. But relationships don't thrive on scorekeeping; they thrive on shared humanity. Pain isn't a contest; it's a chance to say, *"This is hard for both of us. Let's face it together."*

Still, when we're stretched too thin, our instinct is often to protect ourselves. We want our struggle to be seen and validated, so we push for space sometimes without realizing we're crowding out our partners. That's when empathy starts to fade. We stop hearing each other clearly because we're too stuck in our own heads, just trying to get through the moment. And the more we pull inward, the easier it is to miss what our partner might need, too.

Activity: Don't be a "Me Monster"

*One thing I often encourage my clients to do is pause and lean into their partner's struggle **before** bringing up their own. It's not that your feelings don't matter; they do. But when both people are trying to prove who's more exhausted or overwhelmed, connection goes out the window—timing and presence matter. If you want to feel seen, start by seeing them.*

Brian Regan has a hilarious stand-up bit about the "Me Monster." We all know this person, at a party, family dinner, or in a random conversation, who hijacks every story. No matter what you say, they have a bigger, better, more dramatic version ready to go. You had surgery? You say, "I had surgery once," and they fire back, "Oh really? I had triple brain surgery while skydiving, and I performed it myself!" Every story becomes a competition for attention, and the Me Monster always has to win. When you immediately jump in with your own pain right after your partner shares theirs, you become an emotional Me Monster. You steal the spotlight, even if you don't mean to. And just like you'd roll your eyes at that guy at a party, your partner feels dismissed when their pain gets overshadowed. This isn't about ignoring your own needs—it's about creating trust. Let them have the mic. Listen. Soften. When people feel safe and seen, they're far more likely to offer that same space in return. Emotional support isn't a contest; it's a rhythm. Not simultaneous, but shared.

Bottom line: No one wins the "who's struggling more" game. You're on the same team. Let them have their moment. Yours is coming. And when you both lean in instead of away, that's where the real connection begins.

Something I have had to do in my own brain and work on with my wife is the idea of looking at each other when we start competing and stepping away when it feels a little too competitive.

This happened just a few months ago. My son still has rough nights now and then, mostly due to his allergies. Some nights, he wakes up multiple times *before* we've even made it to bed. In our house, we try to avoid having the kids sleep in our bed, so we do what we call a "sleepover" in their rooms. We drag a mattress in, set up camp, and try to get through the night. But let's be clear, this is not the kind of sleepover you remember from childhood. There are no midnight snacks, no silly games. Just coughing, water requests, middle-of-the-night cuddles, and the sound machine working overtime to muffle the chaos.

One of those nights hit hard. I barely slept. But come morning, I stumbled out of the room, half-awake, and asked my wife how *she* slept. She looked at me and said, "Not so great. Belle (our dog) kept me up all night, she missed you."

Every cell in my body wanted to snap. *Really? The dog?* I wanted to rattle off a list of everything I'd just survived: the wake-ups, the coughing fits, the back pain from the floor mattress. But I caught myself. I took a breath. Escalating the pain wouldn't help either of us. So I just listened. I let her vent. And after she felt heard, she asked about my night too. We both got what we needed: empathy, not a scoreboard.

This might hit a nerve, but I promise, it can change the way you think about life with a baby, especially in those early, chaotic months.

Everything changes so fast in the beginning. One minute you're pregnant or waiting, and the next, you're dropped straight into a tornado with no warning. You're dizzy, overwhelmed, and just trying to hang on.

One thing I've had to work on is letting go and not taking life too seriously. In those early days, your goals are simple:

- Keep the baby safe.
- Keep the baby fed.
- Try to survive.

Everything else is the cherry on top. But many people feel like they have to do more to feel calm and in control, especially because this stage of life can feel so uncertain. They see the mess, look at themselves, and panic, thinking it's all going to ruin their baby's well-being. But that's not true. It's just a way of coping with all the chaos around them.

The house doesn't have to be spotless. The laundry can wait. Takeout is your new best friend. Right now, the goal isn't perfection; it's endurance, grace, and rest when you can get it. And when it comes to your relationship, focus on the little things that keep you connected, like a quick hug, a shared cup of coffee, or a simple "I love you" text. It might not be the grand gestures you're used to, but it's enough to remind each other that you're in this together.

The mental noise can get loud, endless to-do lists, intrusive thoughts, guilt, and fear. But try to take a breath and come back to this: You're doing your best. And that is enough.

There will be time for deep cleaning, folded laundry, and dinner parties again. Right now, it's okay to let go, lower the bar, and focus on what you *can* control: safety, love, and presence.

Do One Small Thing

I know I already wrote a whole chapter on self-care, but it bears repeating here, because this is often the moment we need it most. When we are at our end and feeling tired, it is the easiest time for our minds to convince us that we don't matter, and we need to keep pushing forward.

A client recently told me how exhausting hustle culture feels, like no matter how hard you try, it's never enough, and there's always more to do.

Now imagine you feel that with two to four hours of sleep and a screaming baby.

You can't compare yourself to anyone else but who you are today.

Instead of yelling at yourself for how messy or hard life feels right now, cheer for how much you're managing, especially while exhausted and overwhelmed. Both yelling and cheering are loud, but one tears you down, and the other lifts you up. Choose support over self-criticism. You deserve encouragement, not attacks.

And keep it simple. I'm a big believer in small, attainable wins. Whether it's doing the dishes, putting away your clothes, trimming your nails, or taking a shower, any one of those is a victory. Don't overlook it.

Let today's wins stand on their own. Don't let yesterday's unfinished tasks or tomorrow's worries steal their worth. You showed up. You kept going.

Activity: In Hand

As someone who struggles with ADHD and getting things done, I've had to get creative with how I approach daily tasks. Over time, I've developed a tool I call *In Hand*.

The "In Hand" method boils down to four simple questions I ask myself—and that I often share with clients:

1. **Priority:** What *needs* to be done today?
2. **Time:** How long will this actually take?
3. **Energy:** Do I have the physical *and* mental energy for it right now?
4. **Help:** Can I outsource this to my partner, or pay for support (if we can afford it)?

Once you've answered these questions, you can approach a task with more clarity and less pressure—based on *your* current capacity, not some unrealistic ideal.

In-Hand Examples

- **The Clothes in Your Hand**

    I come home from a long day at work, and I need to change. I take off my clothes, and I've got them *in hand*. At that moment, I have three choices: walk them to the hamper, hang them up, or drop them right on the floor. It's a simple moment, but a choice nonetheless. The key is catching that *in-hand* opportunity and doing something manageable with it.

- **The Sink Situation**

   There's a mountain of dishes in the sink. It's overwhelming. But I know the baby bottles and coffee mugs need to be cleaned. That's the *priority*. I set a timer for 10 or 20 minutes, put on music or a podcast (I hear *The Dude Therapist* is fantastic!), and focus on just what's essential. I can do what I can with what I have, or try to conquer the whole mess and burn myself out.

- **The Playroom Paralysis**

   I walk into the kids' playroom and feel that familiar "Where do I even begin?" spiral. Instead of trying to clean it all, I pick a few key zones: the walkway, the couch, the Lego landmines, and clear just those. It's not perfect, but it's progress.

- **The Stench and the Shower**

   I haven't showered in days, and I *need* one. I can ignore it and go to bed…or I can take 5–10 minutes to rinse off and feel a bit more like myself. That's what's *in hand*.

The "In Hand" mindset is about doing *something* instead of nothing. A small action today beats a giant, looming task tomorrow. It's a way to work with your current energy, time, and priorities, *not against them*, so that overwhelm doesn't become paralysis.

This chapter was raw. We explored the nerves that come with sleep deprivation, shifting identity, relationship strain, and the quiet fear that creeps in when the sun goes down. I've lived it. I've cried at the dinner table. I've seen the beauty and pain in clients sitting across from me. But I've also seen healing start with a simple truth: "This is hard." Naming it doesn't fix everything but it's the first step in taking back your power.

Parenting in the early days isn't just hard; it's disorienting. You're trying to function on little sleep, keep your relationship alive, and somehow still recognize yourself in the process. And in that chaos, the little things; one small task, one kind word, one deep breath become lifelines. That's what this chapter was about: giving yourself that grace, teamwork, and one small act of care at a time will carry you through. You don't have to do it all. You just have to keep going.

Now that we've talked about surviving the sleepless trenches, it's time to explore how all of this changes *you*. What happens when you go from "just a guy" to "Dad"? That's up next in *From Dude to Dads*. And after that, we dive into the quiet superpower that often goes unseen but is felt everywhere *Mama Magic*.

6

From Dudes to Dads: The Role of Fatherhood

"Daddies don't cry, only mommies do"

—My daughter, five years old

IN MY YEARS as a father and therapist, one truth has become painfully clear: fatherhood is often overlooked in the parenting conversation. Books, blogs, and support groups tend to focus on mothers, leaving dads with outdated stereotypes and very little guidance. We're expected to show up, provide, maybe toss a football, and keep our feelings in check. But what about the deeper emotional and relational work of being a father? Where is that represented?

This chapter is my attempt to change that. I aim to fill the silence with real stories, honest reflections, and the hard-won truths I wish someone had shared with me before I stepped into fatherhood. That lack of representation and guidance is what eventually pushed me to start posting on social media. I realized that if I was feeling lost, I likely wasn't alone. So, I decided to open up and to be more vulnerable and honest about what it's really like to be a father, the good, the bad, and the ugly. It wasn't easy at first; society doesn't exactly encourage men to talk about their feelings, especially when it comes to parenting. But once I started, I found a community of dads who were all facing similar challenges, all searching for the same kind of understanding and support that I was.

In his book *The Good Son*, Michael Gurian says,[1]

> *"The boy and the man must be raised to see the possibility of self-worth, then meet a few others who provide the vision of a road toward it, then spend a lifetime pursuing that worth through action and relationship. One of the great tragedies in human life is to be born a male and not be guided toward the value of a man."*

We need each other to learn from one another, share, and follow in each other's footsteps.

Being vulnerable and authentic to the experience of fatherhood has been a game changer for me. It's allowed me to connect with other fathers in a way that's real and meaningful, not just on social media but in my everyday life. And it's also made me a better parent and partner, because I'm no longer trying to fit into some mold of what a dad should be. Instead, I'm embracing the full spectrum of what fatherhood can be. This chapter is my way of paying it forward, sharing the lessons I've learned so that other dads don't have to feel like they're in this alone.

The Test

"This is Sparta!"

That iconic line from *300* conjures images of battle-hardened warriors, unflinching courage, and chiseled abs. But beneath the spectacle, there's a deeper message, one that has echoed through generations: to become a man, you must be tested.

Across cultures and history, rites of passage have marked the powerful transition from boyhood to manhood. In Jewish tradition, a Bar Mitzvah symbolizes the acceptance of adult responsibilities within the community. Among the Maasai, boys once proved their strength, courage, and independence by killing a lion. However, today, in the spirit of conservation, this is often replaced with symbolic ceremonies or nonlethal challenges. In Aboriginal Australia, young men embark on a walkabout, journeying alone into the wilderness for weeks or even months, surviving off the land and deepening their spiritual connection to their ancestors. In the Sateré-Mawé tribe of the Brazilian Amazon, boys demonstrate resilience and bravery by enduring the excruciating sting of bullet ants, placing their hands into woven gloves filled with the insects for several minutes without crying out, a trial repeated multiple times before they are recognized as men.

These rituals share a common purpose: transformation. As Michael Gurian writes in *The Wonder of Boys*,[2] "Boys become men in the presence of men who guide, challenge, and initiate them." The journey isn't just about physical endurance; it's about emotional readiness, identity, and belonging. In 300, young Leonidas undergoes his own rite of passage. Alone in the wilderness, armed with nothing but a spear, he faces a wolf. The animal isn't just a threat; it's a symbol of fear, uncertainty, and the weight of future responsibility. Killing the wolf marks his transformation. He returns not just older but changed, capable of leading and protecting. Today, we don't send young men into the forest to fight wolves. But that doesn't mean they don't still exist. Our wolves just look different.

As Sebastian Junger writes in *Tribe*,[3] "Modern society has perfected the art of making people feel unnecessary." Without a clear rite of passage, many boys struggle to find their identity, searching for something, anything, that gives them a sense of purpose and belonging. They search for meaning in silence, unsure where to turn. So, where do young men today find their "wolves"? The challenges are different now but just as real and important. It might be stepping into the role of a father, taking on financial responsibility, or confronting the emotional vulnerability that society has conditioned men to avoid. These are the modern rites of passage, the tests that forge character and strength.

They show up in the moments that demand emotional courage. Becoming a father. Being vulnerable with a partner. Taking responsibility—not just financially but relationally. These moments test us in quieter, but no less significant, ways. They ask: Will you show up? Will you face the fear? Will you let this change you?

Leonidas didn't face the wolf just for his own growth. He did it to prepare himself to lead his people and stand against impossible odds. The journey to manhood is deeply personal, but its impact ripples outward to family, to community, to the world.

Over the last two years, I've worked with countless men in their late twenties to mid-fifties—some single, some stepping into fatherhood—quietly wrestling with the weight of modern masculinity. I've also worked with other men whose children are grown, now faced with redefining their lives and rediscovering their sense of purpose. These are men who have spent their lives navigating the expectations of manhood without ever being given a map. No one ever asked them, "What does being a man mean to you?" They were just thrown into it, expected to figure it out on their own, without guidance or the space to question what feels right and healthy for them.

This work has been incredibly powerful, not just for them, but for me, too. Watching these men face their struggles head-on, their fears, doubts, and the pressures they've carried for so long is inspiring. Each one is confronting his own version of what I call "wolves," the inner battles that have shaped them. And being part of their journey, helping them step into a version of manhood that feels true to who they are, has been one of the most rewarding experiences of my life.

My wolf came in the form of a panic attack.

It was 2 a.m. when I shot awake, overwhelmed by the sense that something was deeply wrong. My face tingled, my heart pounded, and I couldn't catch my breath. I remember stumbling into the living room, collapsing onto the floor, and curling into a ball, hoping the sensation would pass. For half an hour, I lay there, convinced I was dying. Eventually, I cried out. My wife woke up, joined me on the floor, and held me until I finally calmed down.

This was two months into fatherhood. That moment, the fear, the overwhelm, the physical unraveling was my initiation. My version of the wolf.

I can't tell you what was going through my mind that woke me up, but I can give you a little insight into my journey into fatherhood and what it takes to go from a dude to a dad.

Bessel Van Der Kolk puts it so well, "The greatest sources of our suffering are the lies we tell ourselves,"[4] and I was lying to myself that it was all okay and that I was fine. Because deep within, I was screaming in pain, and it had to come out.

I didn't see it coming. I had convinced myself that everything was fine. After all, we had fought hard to get here. My wife and I struggled to become parents, enduring multiple rounds of IVF, each step packed with appointments, needles, and uncertainty. When it finally worked, we held on tight to the hope that this was it—our chance to build the family we'd dreamed of. I was overjoyed and quietly terrified.

I often joke with new dads that moms get nine months to grow into their new role, while dads get about nine seconds. The moment that the baby arrives, we're expected to catch up instantly. Even the most emotionally prepared among us feel blindsided.

If our wives struggle with that massive pivot, we have to give ourselves the grace to adjust as well.

I didn't adjust well at all. Due to the IVF process we had to go through, I became Mr. Do-It-All in my mind to make sure everything went smoothly. Throughout the pregnancy, I tried to be the rock. I paid attention to my wife's mood, her eating, and her sleep. I buried my own emotions beneath the weight of responsibility. I told myself I was being supportive. In reality, I was disappearing.

When labor came, it was smooth, until it wasn't. My daughter's heartbeat suddenly dropped, and in a matter of minutes, everything changed. The room was in chaos. Nurses and doctors scrambled. My wife and daughter were rushed into emergency surgery. And for five endless minutes, I thought I was going to lose everything.

They both came out okay. Healthy. Breathing. Alive. But trauma doesn't leave the room just because the danger passes. It stays. It lingers in your body, your breath, your nervous system. And eventually, it comes out whether you're ready or not.

In Gabor Maté's book, *When the Body Says No*,[5] says so powerfully, "The research literature has identified three factors that universally lead to stress: uncertainty, the lack of information, and the loss of control." And in that moment, I had all three of these factors, and it felt overwhelming. I held it together in the moment until I didn't. I ran to the bathroom, vomited, wiped my face, and went straight into "action mode." Like many men, I pushed it down. That's what we're taught: hold it in, be strong, take care of everyone else.

I wrestle with the instinct to bury my own needs deep down, like I'm some sort of parenting superhero who can handle anything without breaking a sweat. Who wouldn't want to be seen as the rock, the unshakable force holding everything together? But I've learned that strength doesn't mean silence. It doesn't mean pushing through at all costs or pretending I'm fine when I'm unraveling inside. The more I try to play the part of the invincible parent, the more I miss the point. My family doesn't need a superhero. They need *me*—the real, imperfect, sometimes overwhelmed, but fully present version of me.

It's funny how we convince ourselves that strength means silence and that if we just power through and keep our own struggles hidden, we're doing everyone a favor. But that's not what our kids or partners need. They don't need a parent who's always "on" but secretly running on empty. They need someone whole, someone who's honest about their own needs and willing to take care of themselves so they can truly be there for the family. Real strength isn't about pretending everything's fine; it's about acknowledging when it's not, and taking the steps to fix it.

When I finally let go of the idea that I had to be the pillar of strength, I discovered something deeper: vulnerability is its own kind of power. By taking care of myself and not being afraid to admit when I'm struggling, I'm not just setting a good example; I'm showing my family that it's okay to be human. I'm showing them that it's okay to need help, to rest, to feel. That it's not weakness, it's wisdom.

In those early months, I dropped nearly 15 pounds. I was constantly monitoring my wife and our newborn. I was physically present, but emotionally dissociated. And that night on the floor, my body finally said, "Enough."

As Van Der Kolk writes, "As long as you keep secrets and suppress information, you are fundamentally at war with yourself,"[6] I had been at war, trying to be everything for everyone, without admitting I was falling apart.

Open Your Heart

Something I wish someone had said to me years ago is, *Stop being strong; instead, be honest.*

More than a decade ago, I lost my grandmother, one of the most important people in my life. I had support around me, but I didn't let myself feel it. Instead, I focused on my parents' grief, believing that my role was to be steady for them. No one asked me to do that. I just assumed I had to.

Months later, I cracked. While having dinner with my parents, something small triggered a wave of grief. I collapsed onto my mother's lap and sobbed. I didn't need to be the strong one; I needed to be honest.

Recently, my uncle died. As I was getting ready for the funeral, my daughter saw me crying. She asked if I was okay. I told her no and explained why I was feeling sad. And she responded with something that stopped me cold:

"Daddy, you can't cry. Only mommies cry."

That moment is why I needed to write this chapter. The idea that boys and men must suppress their pain is still being passed down, even in our most loving homes.

We need to challenge that story.

In the past few years, I've worked with more men in therapy than ever before, men from all walks of life, each carrying silent weight. They've cried, shouted, and vented. Not once have I seen weakness. I've only seen courage.

Not because I'm a therapist but because I'm a man who knows what it takes to open your heart in a world that tells you to shut it tight.

I've also seen the damage done when vulnerability is met with judgment. In couples therapy, I sometimes hear a partner say, "I want him to open up," followed by, "But I don't want him to become some weak, emotional mess." That contradiction is heartbreaking. It sends a mixed message: be vulnerable but only on terms that feel safe for others.

There's a scene in *Friends* where Rachel encourages Paul (played by Bruce Willis) to open up emotionally. When he finally does, crying for hours, she's visibly uncomfortable. The message is clear: there's a limit to how much vulnerability is socially acceptable from men.

Just because men have feelings doesn't mean they'll fall apart. And even if they do, they still deserve a place to express them without shame. Men need space to let it out. To be raw, honest, and real. Not performatively strong. Just human.

Let them open their hearts. Let them speak without fear. Because when we create space for men to be emotionally true, we don't weaken them, we liberate them.

You Are Enough

There were multiple research studies done in 2010[7] and 2020[8] asking a very simple question: "What is the most important thing to you in your relationship?" The common theme for men was to either be seen or be respected. All men want is to be seen for their efforts and how hard they are working, even if it seems minimal to the people in their lives.

In the months following my panic attack, I felt lost. I didn't know how to show up for my wife or my daughter. I watched them bond through feedings, snuggles, and play, and I stood on the sidelines, unsure of my role and filled with shame. I felt like I was failing.

Around that same time, I got an unexpected call from *The Kelly Clarkson Show*. They wanted me to speak on fatherhood. I said yes, but inside, I was panicking. *Who am I to talk about being a dad?* I felt like an imposter, performing a role I hadn't earned. Sitting on that couch, talking about parenting, I smiled on the outside while silently battling self-doubt.

That experience became a turning point. I realized that unless I confronted that narrative of *You're not enough*, it would eat me alive.

Paternity leave saved me. It gave me the opportunity to confront my biggest challenge, myself, and force it to the surface and show up because I had to, no excuses.

I remember the night before my wife was going back to work, and I spiraled. I was terrified. I imagined everything that could go wrong. I didn't believe I was capable. I had no confidence that I was cut out to be a dad, and maybe all the years of dreaming of this through IVF were all a waste.

I tell fathers all the time: the old rites of passage were meant to challenge you, to push you toward your purpose. For me, this was it. My wolf wasn't in the wilderness. She was wrapped in a swaddle, depending on me for everything.

In those early days of paternity leave, I had to face my fear, my identity loss, and the narrative that I didn't belong. I made mistakes. I cried. I doubted myself. But I kept showing up. And somewhere in that exhausting and beautiful process, I became a father.

Let Them Fail

One of the most powerful tools for fatherhood is something we rarely talk about: the space to fail. One of the reasons paternity leave is such an important step and tool for any dad is the power it gives to moms to trust the process of their partner becoming a father. But too often, that opportunity gets cut short by a phenomenon known as *maternal gatekeeping*, or what some call "The Push Out." It happens when a mother, often unintentionally, takes over parenting tasks out of habit, anxiety, or frustration, leaving little room for her partner to learn and participate.

A few years ago, I was working with a mom:

Harper: *Eli, I am sick and tired of having to do so much for my newborn. I have to feed her, change her, put her to nap and bed, and my husband doesn't help.*

Eli: *I'm so sorry that you're doing all that. Just a simple question: do you ever let him help?*

Harper: *How could I, he doesn't know how to change the diaper right or bathe her well? I can't let him.*

Eli: *So...how about you either include him in the process or step back and see what happens. Pick something low-stakes, like bedtime stories or diaper changes, and step back just a little. Let him fail and learn.*

Fathers grow by doing, and doing means getting it wrong sometimes. We have to let that happen. I know it can be scary to let go when you have been doing such an amazing job. When it comes to raising your kids, it is such a delicate balance of feelings of success and failure.

Like the moment you finally get your kid to sleep. You carefully get on your hands and knees and slowly creep out while holding your breath. One wrong step and the baby wakes up, and who knows how long you'll be stuck back in that rocking chair.

It's a risk you *must* take as a mother and let the father find their path in this crazy world of parenting. You'll be surprised how capable, intuitive, and strong your men are when given the chance to fail with no repercussions.

In the beginning, my wife did so much due to maternity leave and was in such a flow and rhythm to it all that I didn't ever want to mess it up and cause trouble. I felt like a burden if I asked to help or wanted to hold, cuddle, change a diaper...or really do anything. To the dads reading this: **ask to participate**. Don't wait to be invited. Yes, you might put the diaper on backward or overheat the bottle or forget the swaddle trick. That's okay. Your partner made mistakes, too. What matters is that you keep showing up.

And to the moms: **let them**. Let them fail. Let them figure it out. That's how confidence is built.

I'd rather you show up and make some minor mistakes, learn from them, and be a better man and father than not try or do at all. You are such a key factor in your kid's life; don't miss the opportunity given to you. Don't run and hide, embrace the suck, challenge, and moments of parenting by being there and earning your place at the table.

We Listen + We Don't Judge

One of the most significant barriers to connection, especially for men, is the fear of judgment. We've been taught for so long that expressing emotion makes us weak that even when we want to open up, we hesitate. And when we do share, the response we get matters.

I've seen it in therapy time and again: men trying to articulate what they're feeling only to shut down when they sense shame, defensiveness, or misunderstanding. That fear of being labeled "too sensitive" or "too much" can be paralyzing.

I've felt it myself. There have been moments over the last six years of parenting when I've opened up about feeling inadequate or overwhelmed. And sometimes, instead of feeling heard, I felt like my emotions triggered guilt in my wife, like my pain implied she was doing something wrong.

But emotional struggle isn't blame. It's vulnerability.

If we want our partners to share honestly, we have to create space where they can do so safely without criticism, without correction, and without turning their pain into a reflection of our failures.

For men, emotional safety isn't just about being heard; it's about not being punished for feeling deeply. When we feel safe, we speak. When we're judged, we retreat.

So if you want to connect with the man in your life, your partner, your friend, your son start here:

Listen.

Don't correct.

Don't shame.

Let him feel, fully.

Because when a man opens his heart, what he needs most isn't a solution. He needs to know it's still safe to speak.

Addition, Not Subtraction

A few years ago, I sat across from a young dad in the thick of parenting a toddler, with another baby on the way. He was exhausted and overwhelmed.

He told me something that has stuck with me ever since:

> Eli, I used to do so much! "I used to go skiing. I hiked, traveled, and had adventures. I knew who I was. Now...I don't even recognize myself. I love my family, but I miss me."

I stood there for a moment, absorbing the weight of what he was saying. Here was a guy who loved adventure, movement, and independence, and now he felt like he was disappearing under the weight of diapers, sleepless nights, and the weird ability that toddlers have to sense when you're about to sit down and immediately need something.

So many parents feel this way, especially dads. Society tells us that parenthood is this magical, rewarding journey, but no one prepares you for the sense of loss that can come with it. There's this weird grief that sneaks up on you, not for a person, but for yourself. For the person you used to be before you had a tiny, loud, demanding roommate.

And I get it. Before kids, you had time to hit the gym, go on spontaneous road trips, or just *sit in silence*. Now, silence usually means someone is drawing on the walls with a marker, and your "adventures" involve navigating the minefield of LEGOs on your living room floor.

So, I told him, "You're not losing who you are; you're adding to who you've always been."

And that's something every parent needs to hear. *You are not disappearing. You are evolving.*

Think about it. You weren't the same person at 30 that you were at 20. You've evolved through every life stage: relationships, careers, growth, loss. Parenthood is another evolution. Another layer.

And why does that have to be a bad thing?

Yes, your adventures may look different now. Ski trips become sledding lessons. Hikes turn into nature walks with tiny hands collecting rocks. Your adventures aren't gone; they're just shifting.

And sure, some of it is hard. You might miss the independence. You might miss the version of yourself who had energy, certainty, or peace and quiet. But this new version of you?

He's deeper. More grounded. More capable of love than ever before.

You haven't vanished. You've expanded. You are becoming *more*, not less.

Take notice of all that you are building to the already amazing self and appreciate how deep you are becoming as a human.

Appreciating What You're Building

We live in a world that glorifies independence, yet the most fulfilling aspects of life often stem from connection. And right now, you are building something *huge*. You are shaping a little human, teaching them about the world, and helping them grow into decent adults.

Take a moment to appreciate how much you've grown. You have leveled up in ways that your past self couldn't have imagined.

That's not losing yourself. That's *becoming a superhero*.

And yes, it doesn't always feel that way. Some days, you're in survival mode. Some nights, you lie awake wondering if you're doing enough or doing anything right.

You are doing something incredible. *You are not failing. You are becoming.*

So don't give up on yourself. Talk about what you're feeling. Find people who get it. Surround yourself with those who will support you in the tough times and celebrate you in the good times.

Most importantly, know this: *you are not alone.*

Parenting isn't something you're supposed to do in isolation. Your family *needs* you, your partner *needs* you, and yes, we *need* you too.

As Wade Boggs once said, "Anyone can be a father, but it takes someone special to be a dad."

If there's one thing I've learned on this wild journey from going from a *dude* to a *dad*, it's that fatherhood isn't a title you earn the moment your child is born. It's something you grow into.

This chapter was a love letter to dads who are trying their best, whether they're feeling seen or not. But as much as our journey matters, we're not doing this alone. And if we're going to be honest about what it means to step up and show up, we also have to talk about the magic happening right beside us. The quiet, steady, powerful presence of the mothers holding so much, often without recognition.

So now, it's time to shift the focus and honor *her*. The one who often anticipates every need before it's spoken. The one who is learning, unlearning, adapting, breaking, and rebuilding in real time. Let's step into the next chapter and take a deeper look at the strength, wisdom, and beauty of *Mama Magic*.

Notes

1. Michael Gurian, *The Good Son* (Tarcher, 1999) https://openlibrary .org/books/OL16954352M/The_good_son.
2. Michael Gurian, *The Wonder of Boys: What Parents, Mentors, and Educators Can Do to Shape Boys Into Exceptional Men* (Tarcher, 1997).
3. Sebastian Junger, *Tribe: On Homecoming and Belonging* (Harper Collins, 2016).
4. Bessel A. Van Der Kolk, *The Body Keeps the Score: Mind, Brain and Body in the Transformation of Trauma* (Penguin Books, 2014).
5. Gabor Maté, *When the Body Says No: The Cost of Hidden Stress* (Random House, 2019).
6. Bessel Van Der Kolk, *The Body Keeps the Score* (Penguin Books, 2014).
7. Pew Research Center, *The Decline of Marriage and Rise of New Families* (Pew Research Center's Social & Demographic Trends Project, 2010).
8. S. Joel et al., "Machine Learning Uncovers the Most Robust Self-report Predictors of Relationship Quality Across 43 Longitudinal Couples Studies," *Proceedings of the National Academy of Sciences* 117, no. 32 (2020): 19061–19071.

7

Mama Magic

"There's no way to be a perfect mother and a million ways to be a good one"
—Jill Churchill

IN 2019, I was sitting in a small office in a Queens clinic, running on fumes from a 10-hour shift and the exhaustion of having a newborn at home. I was getting through probably eight to twelve clients that day, hoping someone wouldn't show up so I could have a moment to breathe, do my notes, and pee. I didn't know that this day would change my life.

Out of nowhere, every communication channel I had started blowing up, my website, LinkedIn, social media, even my phone. Someone claiming to be a producer from *The Kelly Clarkson Show* wanted to talk about having me on the show in a few days. I assumed it was a scam, but I followed up, just in case.

It was real.

They'd found a story I had shared online about supporting my wife during nighttime breastfeeding. I wasn't the one feeding the baby, but I made a point to show up, stay awake, and support her through those long nights. The show was in its first season and wanted to feature fathers who support mothers. I asked them, "Why me?"

I was shocked and, honestly, a little uncomfortable. I called my wife, barely able to get the words out: Kelly Clarkson wanted to talk to me. But deep down, I instantly thought:

- *I'm not the one who should be recognized—my wife is the one breastfeeding.*
- *I haven't done anything extraordinary—just tried to show up.*
- *She should be on the show with me.*

It showed me something very honest about the view on parenting. When a mother does all the right things, showing up for her kids and living within her power, it's overlooked. But when you have a dad as a supporting actor, he gets notoriety, gets invited to a talk show, and is seen as a saint.

So, this chapter shines a light on mothers and the accolades they deserve.

There's a video called *World's Toughest Job*[1] that you should watch if you want a glimpse into the absurd, beautiful chaos that is motherhood. In it, unsuspecting applicants interview for a fake position titled "Director of Operations." Sounds impressive, right? But as the job description unfolds, their faces drop. The role includes standing or moving all day, no breaks, no vacations, and being available 24/7, even on holidays. You need skills in nursing, culinary arts, psychology, logistics, crisis management, and education. Oh, and there's no salary.

The applicants start to laugh nervously. One person asks, "Is this even legal?" And then the twist hits: this job is already being done by millions of people around the world. It's called *being a mom*. Cue the tears, the stunned expressions, and the sudden urge to call their mothers and say "thank you" a hundred times over.

This video hits because it says what so many of us overlook: moms do *everything*, for free. There's no paycheck, no overtime bonus, no vacation days. Just relentless, behind-the-scenes work powered by love. It's a reminder that being a mom isn't a side role or an extra title; it's a full-time, no-holds-barred, emotionally demanding, physically exhausting, deeply meaningful job. And it's done every day without expecting anything in return.

It's a powerful reminder of just how much mothers carry, often without anyone even noticing.

When I first started dating my wife and things began to get serious, we had one of those classic "deal-breaker" conversations. Some were obvious: no smoking, no cheating. Easy. But then she looked me dead in the eyes and said something I didn't fully understand at the time:

"I hate those dumb wife jokes guys make—especially in front of their wives or behind their backs. Don't be that guy."

Of course, I nodded and agreed. But I didn't really get it…until I became a dad.

Over the last six years of being a dad and seeing all the immeasurable contributions my wife has made in our lives, I have become super sensitive to comments and jokes that men make about moms like:

- They only carried the baby; how hard can that be?
- They complained so much about giving birth, but they had all the good meds. I had to sit there forever, and it was so boring.
- Let the maid take care of it.
- [Insert stupid male humor here]

And I'm not going to go on a whole rant here, but I do have one thing to say to the people who make those tired jokes about their wives or partners being "emotional," "lazy," or "over the top" after having a baby: *shut up.*

Your partner carried your child for nine months. She grew a human being inside her body. That alone deserves honor and respect. Not sarcasm. Not dismissal. Not cheap punchlines. Show up. Step up. And recognize the absolute miracle of what she's done.

Motherhood is like a magical, mystical realm that, as a dad, I'll never fully comprehend. It's this extraordinary world where moms seem to possess a secret superpower, a mix of patience, strength, and a sixth sense that I can only admire from the sidelines. Every day, I'm in awe of the way mothers navigate the endless challenges and joys of parenting, handling it all with a grace that leaves me shaking my head in wonder. Seriously, how do they do it? It's like watching a superhero movie unfold in real life.

Throughout this chapter, we're going to dive into the dual nature of motherhood, whether it be the heavy burden or the incredible power that comes with it. Let's be real, moms are often the default parent. Whether it's the midnight wake-up calls or the constant stream of "Mommy" echoing through the house, moms are on the front lines.

Motherhood isn't just about the endless to-do lists or being the go-to person for everything. It's so much more than the daily grind. Motherhood is about being the embodiment of comfort, calm, and home for your kids. It's the feeling of warmth that only the safe haven of a mother can bring. Robert Browning wasn't wrong when he said about motherhood, "All love begins and ends there." Motherhood is the ultimate expression of love, the kind that's unwavering, unconditional, and deeply rooted in the very core of who a mother is.

So, while we'll talk about the hard stuff, the exhaustion, the mental load, the moments of doubt, let's not forget to celebrate the incredible, powerful love that defines motherhood. It's the kind of love that transforms a house into a home, that soothes fears with just a hug, and that makes all the sacrifices worth it. Motherhood is a tough gig, no doubt, but it's also the most beautiful, impactful role anyone could ever play. And as a dad, I'm just grateful I get to witness it up close every day.

The following are a few stories from my own life that I hope can carry the message home.

1. When my wife had to be pulled into emergency surgery and get an unplanned C-section, there was immediate fear and panic that took over. We felt the urgency flowing through the staff and ripples of intensity in the room. Something I remember very clearly that my wife did, she looked me deep in my eyes and said, "I have to breathe and calm myself down so our baby can be okay." This, to me, is one of the most badass things a mother can do: put herself last for the life of her children, even in the face of fear and distress.

2. There was one day that Max had *that* cough, the kind that makes your stomach clench even though your brain tells you it's probably nothing, but he has a history of allergic reactions, which cause breathing issues. But by late afternoon, it wasn't nothing. His breathing changed, his color shifted, and suddenly we were in go-mode. Everyone has their strengths. In emergencies, I'm usually the one who steps in. I've always had this ability to stay calm when things get intense. Chaos doesn't rattle me; I lock in, assess, and act. It's almost automatic.

   But this time, without a word, my wife said, "I'll take him." Not because she needed to prove anything. Not because I couldn't handle it. But because she *knew* in that deep, unshakable, mama-instinct kind of way that Max needed *her*. That she needed to be the one there. And honestly? That quiet confidence, that willingness to face her fear and discomfort for him, was the strongest thing in the room. She doesn't always *want* to be in those situations. But she shoved her fears aside, packed the diaper bag, grabbed his favorite stuffed animal, and walked out the door with purpose.

   That's not just love. That's bravery.

   Because parenting isn't just about who handles chaos better or who has a steadier hand in the storm, it's about who *shows up*, over and over, even when it's hard, even when it pushes every button and cracks open old anxieties. She did that for Max that night. She showed up fully, flaws and all, because that's what moms do. And while I'm often the calm in the storm, that night, *she* was the strength in the stillness. The soft voice saying, "It's okay, baby," even when she wasn't sure it was. And that? That's the kind of strength that doesn't need fanfare but deserves to be seen.

3. Something I don't say enough, maybe because it's hard to admit, is that I struggle with being alone with the kids for long stretches of time. Not because I don't love them. I do, fiercely. But parenting solo, even just for a few hours, can stretch me in ways I don't always feel equipped for. I get

overwhelmed, overstimulated, and impatient. The noise, the needs, the constant motion, it just…gets to me sometimes. I don't know if that's a "dad" thing or a me thing, maybe both

But then there's my wife.

This past year, especially, while I've been trying to carve out time to write this book, she's been the one clocking the long days. The never-ending snack requests, the sibling fights, the bathroom meltdowns, the cuddles, the messes, the magic. Hours and hours, days, really, just her and the kids.

And here's what amazes me: I've never once heard her complain about it. That doesn't mean it wasn't hard. It was. I know it was. I saw the tired eyes, the deep sighs, the drained patience. But the way she talked about it, the energy she carried was different. She wasn't resentful. She didn't wear it like a burden. She carried it like a badge of honor.

There's a quiet strength in that. Not flashy or loud. But it's the kind of strength that shows up day after day without needing applause. The kind that turns long hours with needy, wild, beautiful kids into something sacred. And me? I'm still learning. Still working on not seeing time with the kids as something to "get through," but something to lean into. Something that stretches me for a reason. She leads by example, reminding me, without saying a word, that this season isn't about perfection or performance. It's about presence. So here's to the moms who carry the hard without needing a trophy.

4. If I had to write a book or give a title to my wife and so many mothers I have worked with/spent time around, it would be "The Art of Overload and Keeping It All Together." The amount moms do daily is insane! They just do it with a smile or even when it's hard, put their head down, and get it done. One of the most vivid examples for me is watching my wife breastfeed our children. It's one of the most awe-inspiring things I've ever witnessed. The ability to *create food* for our babies is an unbelievable act of giving. But as miraculous as it is, breastfeeding is a heavy, often invisible burden. And yet, my wife wanted to do it with both of our kids.

She believed deeply in the power of that connection and what it gave our children. So night after night, I'd wake up, stumble like a zombie into the kids' rooms, and there she'd be: exhausted but calm, eyes heavy with sleep, milk-stained pajamas, messy hair, and still, somehow, radiating peace. There was this quiet pride she carried, like even through the weariness, she knew she was giving something meaningful.

It wasn't glamorous. It wasn't easy. But it was powerful.

That's the magic of motherhood. The behind-the-scenes sacrifices that don't get celebrated nearly enough. The hard, beautiful, thankless moments that add up to something sacred.

The Default Parent

There's a *Family Guy* scene that every parent, especially moms, feels in their *soul*. In it, little Stewie stands by Lois' side while she's clearly busy and starts repeating her name in every variation imaginable: "Mom. Mom. Mom. Mommy. Mama. Ma. Ma. Ma. Mum. Mumma. Mummy...." It goes on and on until Lois, visibly exhausted, finally snaps: "WHAT?!" And Stewie, with perfect comedic timing, just giggles and says, "Hi," and runs off.

It's hilarious, ridiculous, and oddly...accurate. This moment captures that all-too-familiar dynamic of young kids treating their mom like an on-call concierge. It shows how moms get interrupted 47 times in a single hour, often for requests that are completely unnecessary or just plain absurd. ("My sock feels weird!" "Watch me blink!" "Can you pour the milk I'm already holding?" or... "You want to see something cool?")

The constant interruptions. The expectation that moms will be emotionally available—on demand, without question. Being needed 24/7, often for absolutely nothing. It's the endless chorus of "Mom! Look at this!" and "Mommy! I need you!" that wears moms down, not because it's a string of emergencies, but because it *never stops*.

Kids don't have an off switch. They need moms for everything and for nothing, sometimes just to make sure she'll respond. That's the unspoken weight of motherhood. So yeah, Stewie's being a cartoon menace, but what he's tapping into? It's spot-on. No breaks. No boundaries. Just a constant, looping symphony of "Mom. Mama. Mommy…" until she finally cracks; then they giggle, run away, and do it all over again five minutes later.

This happens all the time in my house. I could be sitting right next to my kids—cuddling with them, fully available, and still, they'll yell for *Mom*, who's in another room, to help them with something. And if I dare suggest *I* do it instead? You'd think the world was ending.

Take this moment with my son a few months ago. He loves his blanket—needs it to snuggle, hold, and carry around the house like a little piece of comfort. One afternoon, he yelled, "Mommy, can you please cover me?" I was *right there*. I gently placed the blanket over him and tucked him in like a pro. And he immediately screamed, ripped it off, and cried, "No! I want Mommy to do it!"

I tried reasoning with my three-year-old. I explained that it's the same blanket. Same tuck-in. Same love. But none of that mattered. A few minutes later, my wife came in, laid the same blanket over him in the exact same way, and just like that, *peace was restored*.

There was no difference. Except *Mom* did it.

It's like a form of emotional Chinese water torture: relentless, constant drops of need that eventually wear you down. One request? Fine. Ten? Annoying. A hundred, all day long? That's when even the strongest begin to crack.

This burden is something we dads will not feel as much, as often due to the nature of the connection children have to their mothers. It's such a powerful and beautiful bond, but we don't talk about it enough. As partners and as a society, we need to tune in more. When we understand where moms are mentally and emotionally, we can show up with the love, support, and compassion they truly need.

Most importantly, we need to *step in anyway*.

Even if the request wasn't directed at us.

Even if the kids protest.

Even if it feels easier to stay out of it.

Step in anyway. Because being the default parent shouldn't be a life sentence, especially when there's another capable adult in the house. Just because you're not the one they asked for doesn't mean you're not the one who can help.

You are a fully capable adult. You live in the same house. You can handle snack requests, outfit negotiations, toy drama, and whatever else the kids are firing off that day. This is your opportunity, your *responsibility*, to show your partner that she's not in this alone.

This is how we show up with love. This is how we share the load.

Even if your toddler screams, "But I wanted Mommy!," step in anyway. Let them scream. Let them be disappointed. That moment of frustration will pass. But the message your partner receives when you take initiative? That lasts.

Mental Load

This is a hot topic right now, so let's get full force into this idea. Mental load is the concept of the overwhelming tabs, to-do lists, school schedules, after-school schedules, playdates, what's for dinner, work, taking care of the house, and who knows what else flying around someone's brain at all times.

It's interesting to reflect on this as a father. Something I didn't dive into fully in the fatherhood chapter is that, yes, dads carry mental load too. But often, it looks different.

For many men, the mental load tends to revolve around big-picture concerns: finances, safety, future planning, career pressure. It takes up a lot of mental space, but it's not usually swirling around all day, every day, in the same way.

For many moms, the load is *constant*. It's the birthday gift that needs to be ordered, the pediatrician appointment that needs rescheduling, the snacks for school, the text they forgot to answer, and the emotional temperature of every family member in the house. It's *all the things, all the time*. And juggling it can feel like holding a stack of fragile glass plates, so when someone adds just *one* more thing, everything threatens to crash to the floor.

Psychologist Susan David talks about this in her influential book *Emotional Agility*, where she describes two kinds of people: *brooders* and *bottlers*. Brooders stew in their stress, going over the same anxieties again and again. Bottlers push their emotions down and move on or implode. She says, "Brooders stew in their misery, endlessly stirring the pot around, and around, and around. Brooders can't let go, and they struggle to compartmentalize as they obsess over a hurt, a perceived failure, a shortcoming, or an anxiety."[2]

So what does that mean in real life? It means your partner may not be "just stressed," she's in a mental feedback loop, replaying things over and over because she feels responsible for *everything*. And that kind of stress isn't just exhausting, it's isolating.

So, what can we do about it?

- As partners, we need to be *actively* aware of what our partners are carrying—not just the visible tasks, but the invisible weight behind them. That takes intention. That takes focus. That takes actually seeing your partner's life, not just your own.
- When you go through the check-in activity from earlier in this book, don't just listen—*step up*. Offer to take on more than what's "normal" for you. Take ownership of the joint life you're building. Take tasks off their plate without needing to be asked. And when you *are* asked, don't make a fuss. Don't roll your eyes. Just do it.
- Ask them! Regularly check in and ask: "What can I take off your plate today?"

If your partner's brain feels like a hamster wheel spinning full speed, don't just cheer her on from the sidelines. *Get in the wheel with her*. Or better yet, help her slow it down.

Because the mental load? It's not a "her" problem. It's a shared problem, and it deserves a shared solution.

You Can't Compare

This part might ruffle some feathers but it's too important to skip.

Stop trying to quantify the efforts of each other.

The tallying, the comparison, the "who did more today" contest, it's a dead end. When we compare efforts, we diminish them. We turn meaningful contributions into math problems when what they really need is acknowledgment.

Let it go.

Stop trying to make it equal. Just *see* the effort. Appreciate it. Say thank you.

Because whether it's one thing or twenty, to the person doing it, it matters.

Now, on the flip side, this is to all the moms out there (please stay with me):

Sometimes, in the exhaustion and overwhelm, the commentary can shift from venting to cutting.

- "I birthed these kids—you should be doing everything you can to repay me."
- "I breastfed for a year and a half. I've made plenty of effort."
- "I changed 17 diapers today—you owe me."

And listen, I get it. Truly. The work you're doing is immense, exhausting, often invisible, and rarely appreciated the way it should be. You're carrying a weight that's hard to describe, let alone measure.

But when those truths are turned into weapons, when they're used to shame or guilt your partner, they can start to erode connection. They can make the person beside you feel small, even when they're trying their best.

So let me say this to *both* partners:

Everyone needs to stop comparing.

It doesn't matter who made more money today, who was home longer with the kids, or who endured more meltdowns. This isn't a competition. It's a family. And every role-played in that family matters.

Share your needs. Speak your truth. And if you're on the receiving end of that honesty, give them grace for even asking. Respond with kindness, not defensiveness. That's how we stay on the same team.

See the Effort

One thought has been with me since the moment I started writing this book:

The love of my life created life.

Let that sink in for a second.

In the hustle of everyday parenting with snacks, tantrums, laundry, and carpool, we rarely pause to acknowledge the extraordinary. We're racing through routines, checking boxes, and trying not to lose our minds. But if you take just a moment to see it, to *feel* it, you'll notice something powerful:

Your partner brought life into this world. That's not small. That's not ordinary. That's sacred.

As someone who has been through IVF and witnessed the emotional and physical toll it takes just to get to the starting line, I've gained a deep appreciation for what it means to carry, deliver, and raise a child. It's a privilege wrapped in exhaustion—a burden filled with beauty.

As Lisa Marshal said, "Labor and delivery is measured in hours. Birth is a moment. Being a parent is the rest of your life."[3]

So what can you do to honor that? It doesn't take a grand gesture. Just a few simple, intentional words:

"Thank You."

"I appreciate all you did for us today."

"You mean everything to me."

"What do you need for yourself today?"

"What's my role today?"

These are the words I try to live by, especially since our second child was born and I finally understood what it meant to truly *communicate about needs*, not just tasks. Not just logistics. *Needs.*

When your partner feels seen, she doesn't have to carry her load with resentment. She can carry it with love because someone noticed. Because someone cared enough to ask.

Your presence, your acknowledgment, your *words* matter. So use them. And use them often.

There's a phrase that's been echoing through parenting spaces—on blogs, in therapy sessions, across Instagram posts—and it's one we need to take seriously:

"Who mothers the mother?"

It's a question that cuts straight to the heart of modern motherhood.

So, who is taking care of a mother if she can't mother herself?

YOU!

We don't have to wait for Mother's Day to pamper, appreciate, or support them. Showing up for the mother of your child can be a *regular rhythm*, not a once-a-year gesture. It's not about big displays, it's about *intentional action*.

- Bring her coffee without being asked.
- Take the kids out so she can nap in silence.
- Handle the bedtime routine even if it's "her night."
- Ask, "How are *you* doing?" and really listen.

It's not complicated. It's consistent.

When a mom feels truly supported, she breathes deeper. She moves through her day with a little more ease. She feels like she's not alone in carrying the weight of the family.

So if you're partnered with a mom who's running at full speed, seeming like she has it all together: *she probably needs someone to hold her the most.*

Not because she's weak.

But because she's been strong for everyone else, for far too long.

Mothers are often the unsung heroes of the home, not because we don't value them but because their magic becomes so ingrained in daily life that we forget to stop and *see* it.

Their patience, their presence, their unwavering dedication, it's the invisible glue that keeps everything from falling apart. But that magic? It's not limitless. It needs replenishment. It needs recognition. And it deserves reverence.

If you're a partner, this is your call to action. Not to be perfect, not to fix everything, but to show up with presence and love. To be the teammate she deserves.

And if you're a mother reading this: I see you. You are doing more than enough. You are the magic your family relies on. You deserve rest, joy, connection, and support that doesn't require asking.

Motherhood is breathtaking in its strength and exhausting in its demands. Let's stop letting it go unseen. Let's honor it. Let's share the load. Let's make sure the ones who make the world go round never feel like they're doing it alone.

When we think about all that mothers carry, the mental load, the invisible labor, the emotional glue, it becomes even clearer that communication isn't just helpful in a relationship; it's *essential*. Because love, as powerful as it is, doesn't read minds.

We can't support one another, truly support, without learning how to talk about what's happening *underneath* the surface. And if we want to show up for each other not just as co-parents but as partners, we need to build bridges between us, one honest conversation at a time.

This next chapter is where we go there.

Notes

1. American Greetings, *The World's Toughest Job* [Video] (YouTube, 2014).
2. Susan David, *Emotional Agility* (Avery, 2016).
3. Lisa Marshall, *Becoming a Dad: The First-Time Dad's Guide to Pregnancy Preparation (101 Tips for Expectant Dads)* (Independently Published, 2019).

8

Pillow Talk 2.0

"Kind words can be short and easy to speak, but their echoes are truly endless."

—Mother Teresa

HAVE YOU EVER experienced the "joy" of being woken up at 3 a.m. by a screaming child? If not, let me set the scene: it fills the house, rattles your nerves, and jolts you from sleep with all the grace of a fire alarm. About a year ago, I found myself in just that situation. As any sleep-deprived parent might, I chose the time-honored strategy of pretending to be asleep. I figured it was probably just a bad dream and if I lay still long enough, the cries might fade.

Spoiler alert: they didn't. Ten minutes later, the urgent cries of "Daddy! Daddy!" were still echoing down the hallway.

When you imagined your future children sweetly calling your name, you probably didn't expect it to sound more like a fire drill than a lullaby. What no one tells you is that for the next two decades, you'll hear your name shouted, whined, and screamed, often before you've had your first sip of coffee.

So, there I was at 3 a.m., finally dragging myself out of bed like a zombie to investigate the chaos. Why was she screaming? Because, in her mind, it was morning. She insisted the sun was up, a bold claim considering the moon was still glowing outside her window. Normally, I'd admire her creativity and maybe even play along, but it was 3 a.m. Creativity has limits.

What followed was an unexpectedly philosophical conversation about "daytime." Standing in the dark, I tried to explain that it wasn't morning because the sun wasn't up, despite my daughter's firm belief that it was. I pointed to the window, gestured at the moon, and mentioned that even animals were still asleep. She looked at me with crossed arms, raised eyebrows, and delivered her argument: "I'm awake, so the day is awake."

I'll give her credit; she made her case with confidence. You'd think reasoning with a four-year-old would be easy, but I was outmatched. After a few minutes that felt like hours, I got her back into bed. I hadn't convinced her, but I had earned a brief moment of silence. I tiptoed back to my room, praying for sleep, but naturally, my brain had other plans.

Back in bed, too annoyed to fall asleep, I grabbed my journal and started writing. As I recounted the whole absurd ordeal, what struck me most wasn't the time or the exhaustion; it was her honesty. At 3 a.m., she had no filter, no second-guessing. She wanted to talk, so she did. No fear of saying the wrong thing. No hesitation.

Somewhere along the way, we lose that ability. We're taught to be quiet, to avoid bothering others, to read the room before speaking. We start suppressing our thoughts, softening our truths, and avoiding anything that might cause conflict. But what if we didn't? Too often, we get stuck trying to say the "right" thing and end up saying nothing at all.

As much as I didn't appreciate the 3 a.m. wake-up call, it left me thinking: what if we spoke more like that? What if we stopped worrying about being perfect and started focusing on being present? Maybe it's time we unlearn some of the unhealthy rules we've absorbed and rediscover the art of simply talking.

This chapter dives into one of the most common challenges I see in relationships: communication breakdown. I've worked with countless couples who love each other deeply but still miss the mark because they lack the tools and language to truly connect. As Oscar Wilde said, "Ultimately, the bond of all companionship, whether in marriage or in friendship, is conversation." At the end of the day, it all comes down to connection.

I often compare couples to a PC and a Mac. At their core, they're both computers—designed to connect, process, and create, but they operate differently. What's intuitive for one might seem confusing or frustrating to the other. It's not that one is better than the other; they're simply built with different systems.

Relationships work the same way. Two people can share similar values, such as love, connection, and family, yet still process emotions, handle conflict, and communicate in totally different ways. Without awareness of how your partner "runs," even the clearest message can be misunderstood.

It's not about fixing your partner. It's about learning their system. When we understand how our partner thinks, feels, and responds, we stop talking past each other and start truly connecting.

When I was six or seven, I thought I had life all figured out. One morning, I bounded down the stairs and walked straight up to my mom, full of energy and what I believed was profound insight.

"Mom," I said, dead serious, "I love life so much."

She stopped in her tracks, eyes wide, clearly moved. Her face softened into a look of emotional awe, and I was thoroughly confused. "Mom, why are you crying?" I asked. "I'm just talking about the cereal."

I had been referring to my favorite breakfast, Life cereal, not the broader existential wonder of being alive. But to her, those three words, "I love life," meant something far deeper.

That moment stuck with me. It taught me something crucial: our words don't just carry meaning; we project meaning onto them based on how we hear them. Communication isn't just about what's said; it's about how it's received. Even a light comment can land heavily if the listener interprets it differently from how we intended.

Super-Communicate

Let's shift gears from cereal wisdom to something more structured: the anatomy of everyday communication. In nearly every conversation, especially in relationships, we're often speaking *past* each other without realizing it. That's not because we don't care, but because we're having *different types* of conversations entirely.

Author Charles Duhigg[1] breaks down conversation into three fundamental questions that shape most of our interactions:

- What is this all about?
- How do we feel?
- Who are we?

These categories sound simple, but they carry immense weight. Whether we're discussing dinner plans or school choices for our kids, we're often unknowingly bouncing between different focuses. And when those focuses don't match, miscommunication and conflict arise—not because of malice but because of a mismatch.

What Is This All About

This includes the decision-making and logistical conversations.

How Do We Feel

This includes the emotional conversations.

Who Are We

A study in 1997 by a neuroscientist, Mathew Lieberman found that 70% of our conversations fall within the confines of this question, which is the social mindset.

If you remember from Chapter 2, "The Holy Trinity," we met Alani and Cooper, partners who deeply love one another but constantly clash over parenting decisions. Whether it was school selection or mealtime dynamics, their arguments weren't just about logistics or emotions. They were speaking two different conversational languages.

When discussing mealtime:

Cooper: *I want to spend more time with you and the kiddo.*

Alani: *We need to get things moving, she needs to eat a certain amount, and I have to clean up. there is no time for chitchat and hanging out.*

When discussing schools:

Cooper: *Public schools are a wonderful place for her social game, they're full of diversity, and they're free, which means we can do more as a family together (a new apartment, trips, and time together).*

Alani: *I need her to be in a private school so she can get into an Ivy League college.*

Both were passionate and sincere. But they weren't having the *same conversation*. Cooper was speaking emotionally about connection and presence. Alani was speaking logistically about outcomes and planning. Neither was wrong. But they were mismatched.

That's where the **Matching Principle** comes in: the ability to recognize what *type* of conversation your partner is having and shift your focus to meet them there. When you tune into their emotional or logistical wavelength rather than doubling down on your own, you create a space where both of you feel seen and heard.

Miscommunication often stems not from bad intentions but from not realizing you're solving different "puzzles" in the same moment. When we ask ourselves, "Are we speaking the same language?" and then pause to clarify, it can transform the tone, direction, and outcome of a conversation.

These are four basic questions of healthy conversations:

- What kind of conversation is this?
- What are the goals?
- What are you both feeling?
- Are identities important to the conversation?

Let's break each one down with real-world examples.

What Kind of Conversation Is This?

Before you can truly connect, you need to know what type of "game" you're playing. Is this a strategy talk, an emotional check-in, or a moment of deeper identity exploration? Getting aligned early on avoids misfires and assumptions.

Think of it like a football team in a huddle. The quarterback doesn't just start the play; he makes sure everyone knows *what* play they're running. If even one player misses the memo, the entire play can fall apart. The same goes for relationships. A quick check-in can make a world of difference.

Here are some examples:

- One of you wants to relax by the pool. The other has a jam-packed itinerary of museums, hikes, and 6 a.m. wakeups.
  - o Huddle moment: "Before we book anything, let's align on expectations, chill vibes or Type-A dream trip?"
- One of you believes in natural consequences. The other is ready to ground your kid for a month because they rolled their eyes.
  - o Huddle moment: "Let's touch base on how we want to discipline, before we both become 'the bad cop' in different ways."
- One of you sends a flirty text and assumes that means sex is on the table. The other sees it as playful but has no intention beyond that.
  - o Huddle moment: "Let's check in on how we're reading signals. Flirting is great, but let's stay clear on what we both want."

These mini "huddles" create clarity before conflict has a chance to fester. They're small, intentional moments that create big results in emotional connection.

What Are the Goals?

Once you've figured out what kind of conversation you're having, the next step is to get clear on the outcome you're both hoping for. Just like in football, once the play is called, the team knows where the ball should go. Without that shared vision, the result is often miscommunication, tension, or emotional fumbles.

In relationships, this means asking "What's the purpose of this conversation?" Are we trying to solve a problem? Vent? Reconnect? Clarifying the goal prevents the all-too-common experience of talking past each other and can stop a small spark of frustration from becoming a full-blown fire.

Here are a few examples:

- *Conversation:* "Hey, I'm feeling overwhelmed and want to figure out a better way to split the house stuff."
  Goal: Find a more balanced system, not attack or blame.
- *Conversation:* "I want us to feel more united when we handle tantrums. Can we talk about our approaches?"
  Goal: Create a parenting game plan, not decide who's the better parent.
- *Conversation:* "Lately I've been feeling a little disconnected and I miss us. Can we talk?"
  Goal: Reconnect, not accuse or rehash every past argument.

When couples don't know the goal of a conversation or assume different ones, they often walk away feeling unseen or misunderstood. But when the purpose is clear, even hard discussions can turn into productive, connecting moments.

What Are You Both Feeling?

So far, we've covered the structure and the strategy, but don't forget the heart. Conversations aren't just logistical check-ins; they're emotional exchanges. And often, it's not *what* we say but *how* we show up for each other's feelings that makes the difference.

Slowing down to acknowledge your partner's emotional state builds safety and trust. One of the simplest and most powerful tools in communication is validation. It doesn't mean you agree with everything your partner is saying; it just means you're acknowledging that their feelings are real and worth caring about.

Validation sounds like:

"I see that this is important to you."

"That must feel so frustrating."

"I get why you're feeling this way."

What Version of Me Do You Need Right Now?

One of the simplest and most overlooked ways to improve communication is by asking your partner what they need from you in the moment.

When I work with couples trying to rebuild trust and deepen their emotional connection, I often suggest they ask two core questions during important conversations:

- "Do you need me to just listen, or would you like advice?"
- "What role do you want me to play in this conversation?"

Each conversation carries a different emotional charge. Some moments call for quiet support, others for problem-solving or reassurance. But if we assume what's needed instead of asking, we risk showing up with the wrong energy, leading to more frustration and missed connections.

When in doubt, ask. Be curious. Your willingness to check in rather than assume can shift the entire tone of your relationship.

This practice helps eliminate guesswork and prevents the classic communication misfires where one partner is venting and the other jumps in to fix, unintentionally shutting them down. By actively checking in and letting your partner set the tone, you create space for emotional safety and clarity, two cornerstones of meaningful connection.

The Sacred Space

Now that we've covered some foundational communication skills, it's time to talk about the one element that makes it all work: safety.

Emotional safety is the cornerstone of connection. It's what allows both partners to speak honestly, listen openly, and navigate hard conversations without fear of rejection or judgment. But the phrase "safe space" has been tossed around so much in recent years that it's lost its meaning. So let's redefine it clearly and practically.

Here's a simple formula I use:

$$Mindset + Time + Place + Reassurance = Safety$$

Mindset is a clear headspace and plan of action.

Time is the space to land your conversation.

Place is about the physical and context of a situation.

Reassurance is the confidence in each other to keep things calm, collected, and focused.

Mindset

A safe conversation starts with the right mindset. That means being mentally and emotionally available, not distracted, stressed, or preoccupied.

Imagine this: *Ava has spent the day managing the household, exhausted and maxed out. Ian walks in the door full of energy, eager to share every detail about his day. Without checking in, he launches into conversation. Ava, understandably distant and overwhelmed, responds flatly. Ian feels rejected. Frustration builds.*

What went wrong?

Not the love. Not the content. Just the timing and delivery.

This could've gone differently if Ian had asked one simple question:

"Hey love, do you have a few minutes? I really want to tell you about something."

That pause, the check-in, is everything. It gives Ava a chance to get grounded and gives Ian a chance to set a collaborative tone instead of creating friction.

Being thoughtful about *how* you enter a conversation can radically change *what* happens during it.

I have seen this solve so many struggles between unbelievably loving and compatible people in a relationship. When they start making the time to speak and make sure the coast is clear to chat with their loved ones, the difference in connection is so palpable.

When it comes to communication, we need to make sure it works for everyone who is involved, because if one of you is off or not fully there, it will immediately ripple throughout the conversation and cause a ticking time bomb of it all exploding and falling apart.

Tip #1: If You Want a Safe Space, Ask for It First

You might be ready to talk, but that doesn't mean your partner is. Set the tone by asking for permission to enter their space, emotionally and mentally. Just like you teach your kids not to interrupt, we need to practice that same courtesy in our adult relationships.

For example, I can't count how many times my kids burst into a conversation between my wife and me with "Mommy!" or "Daddy!" totally unaware of the dynamic already in progress. We teach them to pause, wait, and ask. That same emotional awareness is critical for adults, too.

Before diving into a serious or vulnerable discussion, ask:

> *"Can I talk to you for a minute?"*
> *"Is this a good time?"*
> *"Are you in a space to hear something important?"*

You're not asking for permission to matter; you're asking for permission to be heard well.

Time + Place

We've all heard the saying "Timing is everything." When it comes to communication in a relationship, it's not just timing; it's also **setting**. The emotional and physical space you choose can determine whether your conversation brings connection or conflict.

The Right Time

Let's talk timing first. Here's a story I heard early in my career:

> Jane told me, *"I don't know why my husband's so annoyed at me. We were having sex, really connected and I casually brought up our kid's school schedule for the next day. The energy shifted immediately, and he got upset. I haven't heard from him since. Was it really that bad?"*

As a younger therapist, I wasn't sure what to say. But now? I'd tell Jane this:

> **Yes, it really was that bad.** Not because her concern wasn't valid, but because the *timing* completely missed the mark.

It wasn't the topic; it was the shift. During an intimate moment, abruptly pivoting to logistics can feel like an emotional shutdown. If Jane had waited five or ten minutes, that same conversation might have gone beautifully. But in that moment, it felt like rejection.

Timing isn't about censorship, it's about *respect*. Respect for the emotional space your partner is in, and the kind of connection the moment is meant to hold.

The Right Place

Now, let's talk space.

Where you have your conversations matters just as much as when. I see it all the time: serious conversations unfolding in public settings, with kids around, or even in front of extended family. That lack of intentional space can cause tension, misunderstanding, or discomfort.

When you are:

- *In a public setting:* Find a quieter space, or hit pause. Say, "Let's revisit this when we're home so I can focus on you."
- *Around family:* Step into another room or take a walk. Your personal business deserves privacy.
- *Around your kids:* If a disagreement surfaces in front of them, be civil—and make sure they also witness resolution. Conflict isn't inherently harmful. Watching parents fight *and* make up teaches emotional resilience.

Here's a story my mom shared when I first started dating:

"Growing up, I never saw my parents fight. So when I had my first argument with your dad, I thought we were headed for divorce."

Meanwhile, my dad had watched his parents argue all the time and saw it as normal. Two people. Two different blueprints. Both are valid, but neither complete.

It's not about hiding your conflict, it's about modeling *healthy* conflict. If your kids see arguments, let them also see repair. Let them watch love stretch and stay.

Reassurance

You might be thinking:

"What if it's never a good time to talk?"

No one has to be forced to talk right now…but you do have to talk at some point.

Healthy communication isn't about forcing conversations; it's about making space for them.

Setting boundaries is crucial. If you're overwhelmed, overstimulated, or simply not in the right headspace to connect, you're allowed to hit pause. But, and this is key, you also need to provide a *clear and caring follow-up*. When we give our partner a "when" or "how," we're not shutting them out. We're inviting them in…just not yet.

Here are some real-life examples of how to set that boundary *without* creating distance:

- "Hey babe, I would love to talk to you, but I am just coming out of a meeting and my mind is in a million places. Can you text me the topic, and I'll circle back after the kids are asleep?"
- "I'm so glad you want to chat. I'm headed to school pickup now—can we talk in the car or when I get back?"
- "Hey cutie, I'm in a funk. The kids have worn me down today, and I need 10–15 minutes to reset so I can be present with you."
- "That sounds important, but I am trying to focus on not burning dinner. Can we talk once we're sitting down at the table?"

Each of these examples shares one thing: *reassurance*. They say, "I hear you, I care, and I will show up for you, just not this second."

These small moments of clarity can make or break communication. When we assume our partner's timing and capacity, we risk disconnection. But when we check in, set clear expectations, and commit to revisiting the conversation, we preserve trust and emotional safety.

Feeling safe to talk openly starts with creating the right space, one where both people feel respected and ready to connect.

Even something as simple as "Hey, is now a good time?" can shift the tone entirely. It shows respect. It shows intention. It shows love. When you build that kind of trust, communication feels less like a battle and more like a team effort.

Power of Clarity

A major cause of communication breakdowns isn't the message itself—it's the clarity behind it. It's not what you say, it's how you say it. And it's whether the person you're talking to actually understands what you mean.

Years ago in a training, I heard a simple acronym that stuck with me:

Communication should be HOT—Honest, Open, and Two-Way.

It sounds basic, but it's incredibly powerful.

In Chapter 2, I introduced the concept of naïve realism, the belief that we see the world as it truly is and anyone who disagrees is just wrong, uninformed, or biased.

Let me be blunt: that mindset is toxic in a relationship.

You cannot communicate effectively if you believe your view is the only "correct" one. Your partner has a whole world of context, emotion, and experience that shapes their perspective—just like you do. If you ignore that, you're not communicating. You're broadcasting.

Why Context Changes Everything

Let's say I'm in another room and hear one of my kids crying. I walk in to see my son screaming, red-faced and upset. My first instinct is to turn to my daughter:

"What happened? What did you do to him?"

But if I pause and ask, I might discover that my son grabbed a toy from her, and when she calmly took it back, he lost it. Suddenly, the narrative shifts. I had only half the picture, and my assumption could have led to an unfair accusation.

We do this in adult relationships too.

Maybe your partner let your kid snack on something "off-limits" right before dinner. Instead of jumping in with "Why would you do that?!," try this:

"Hey, I noticed she had a snack. Was she super hungry, or was something going on?"

Curiosity invites conversation. Assumptions shut it down.

When you feel the urge to correct, criticize, or question your partner's judgment, pause. Take a breath. Ask for the full picture. Not everything needs to be a confrontation. Some things just need clarity.

Activity: Full Communication

When I work with couples who struggle to express themselves clearly, I often introduce a deceptively simple practice: **say the full thing.**
    Don't hint.
    Don't assume your partner can read between the lines.
    Don't give the short version and expect them to "get it."
    Say the whole thing—your thought, your why, your request, and what it would mean to you.
    Here are a few examples I offer couples in session:

- *"Hey love, can you please handle the dishes right now? It would help me so much, I still have emails to answer, and I'm feeling overwhelmed."*
- *"I'd love to go to brunch on Sunday. It's my favorite meal, and the timing works well for the kids. That way, we're not rushed for the rest of the day."*
- *"I was thinking of planning a little adventure with the kids in two weeks. I've been missing quality time with them and want to do something active and fun."*
- *"I really need a walk after bedtime. I've been stuck in the house all day and need some air and movement to decompress. Can you do cleanup while I'm out? That would mean a lot."*
- *"Hey babe, I have about 20 minutes of work left. If you can handle the kids, I'll be free and fully present after. Can we tag-team this?"*

In all of these, you're giving your partner clarity, not just about what you want, but why it matters. You're painting the full picture so they can meet you in it. Your partner isn't a mind reader, so express it all. Don't leave anything to guessing or expecting your partner to connect all the dots you have in your own mind.
    And yes, I've had clients say, "But that's a lot to process."
    Okay, but it's a lot more to process when your needs are unmet, resentment builds, and no one knows why.
    When you speak clearly, you give your relationship the gift of understanding and the space to grow from it.

Don't Read Between the Lines…Ask

We've all been told, "Curiosity killed the cat," but in relationships? *Curiosity is the thing that keeps the connection alive.*

Too often, we try to "read" our partner: guessing their mood, intentions, or feelings instead of just asking. We assume. We fill in blanks. We write stories in our heads. And those stories? They're usually wrong.

I hear this all the time in therapy:

- "How am I supposed to know what they're feeling?"
- "They never say what they actually mean."
- "He doesn't express himself—I can't read his mind!"

And my response is always the same: *then stop trying to read minds—ask questions.*

When you lead with curiosity, it tells your partner, "I care about you. I care enough not to just assume. I want to understand your world."

One powerful tool here is what Charles Duhigg calls *emotional contagion.*[2] It's the ability to lock in with someone's emotions through questions, empathy, and focus to connect to them on a deeper level and the power emotions have on the people we are talking to.

Curiosity is a generous act.

It shifts the spotlight off of your assumptions and onto your partner's reality.

Ask things like:

- "Hey, what's coming up for you right now?"
- "Can you tell me more about how you're feeling?"
- "What would feel supportive to you in this moment?"

These are small questions with big impact.

Because when you stop reading between the lines and start asking, you move from confusion to clarity, from frustration to compassion, and from disconnection to authentic connection.

Respond Don't React

Over the last few years, I have been getting a bit obsessed with Viktor Frankl. His view on life, struggle, and the ability to find that inner strength we all have is something that moves me on so many levels. He has been quoted as saying, "Between stimulus and response there is space. In that space is our power to choose our response, In our response lies our growth and our freedom."[3]

Let me tell you about Peter, a client I worked with a few years back. He was a good guy, a deeply caring husband and father, but he was caught in a frustrating cycle. He would come into session upset, confused, and heartbroken by how his conversations with his wife and kids kept spiraling. "I'm not yelling," he'd say. "I'm just answering them. I'm just talking!"

But what Peter couldn't yet see was that he wasn't responding; he was reacting.

When we're emotionally flooded, tired, triggered, or running on empty, we often move fast. We fire back words before we even know what we're trying to say. We try to protect ourselves, to win the moment, to unload something building inside us. And in doing that, we often hurt the people we care about most.

So I asked Peter to try one simple thing: pause for 5 to 10 seconds before responding.

That's it.

Not forever. Just long enough to take a breath, get back into his body, and give himself a moment of choice.

At first, he hated the suggestion. "What's 10 seconds gonna do?" he asked.

But week by week, he practiced. And you know what happened? His reactions softened. His wife stopped bracing for blow-ups. Conversations slowed down. He began to *respond* with more clarity, compassion, and control.

This shift is something I call getting out of "Flash Mode." When I'm there, I'm a tornado of expressions. No filter. No pause. And even if I mean well, my words often come out sharp, messy, or misaligned. That's when I hurt people I never intended to. That's when good intentions get lost in bad delivery.

But a pause? A pause gives us the power to *choose* how we show up. And that power can change everything.

Next up, we're diving into conflict where things get real and spicy. Because as much as we'd like to avoid it, *conflict is part of every relationship*. The good news? It doesn't have to tear you apart. In the next chapter, I'll show you how it can bring you closer, if you know how to fight well.

No matter how much you love each other, you're going to disagree. You're going to misread each other. You'll get tired, frustrated, or triggered, and the conversation will turn from connection to collision. That's not a failure, it's a human relationship.

But here's the truth most of us don't learn growing up: conflict isn't the problem. *How we handle conflict is the problem.*

Do we escalate or stay curious?

Do we go for the jugular or reach for understanding?

Do we shut down or stay present even when it's uncomfortable?

This next chapter isn't about avoiding arguments or turning every disagreement into a rom-com moment. It's about equipping you with the tools to show up when things get hard. To speak with intention, even when emotions run high. To learn that sometimes, *the way you fight is more important than what you're fighting about.*

So take a breath. We're about to enter the arena not to win but to grow.

So, buckle up, it's about to get spicy!

Notes

1. Charles Duhigg, *Supercommunicators: How to Unlock the Secret Language of Connection* (Random House Large Print Publishing, 2024).
2. ibid.
3. Stephen R. Covey, *The 7 Habits of Highly Effective People*, 2nd ed. (Pocket Books, 2004).

9

Love and War

"Peace cannot be kept by force; it can only be achieved by understanding."
—Albert Einstein

IN THE DEAD of night on February 24, 1989, over the Pacific Ocean, just minutes after takeoff from Honolulu, United Airlines Flight 811 was a picture of routine. Passengers settled in for the long haul to Sydney, flight attendants secured the cabin, and pilots guided the massive Boeing 747 through a standard climb. Then, in an instant, chaos erupted.

A deafening explosion ripped through the aircraft as the forward cargo door failed, tearing a massive hole into the plane. The sudden decompression was violent and immediate. Rows of seats, occupied just seconds earlier, were ripped from the cabin, ejected into the freezing darkness of the night sky. Nine lives were lost at that moment.

Alarms blared. The cockpit instruments flashed red. Wind roared through the gaping hole in the fuselage, and oxygen masks dangled uselessly for those who were now gasping for breath. The aircraft, wounded and unstable, shuddered violently. Every second counted.

What happened next was a masterclass in calm under pressure. Captain David Cronin, a seasoned pilot on his final flight before retirement, along with his crew, didn't panic. Years of training and crisis simulations kicked in. Despite the noise, confusion, and damage, they stayed focused. The aircraft was losing fuel and systems were failing, but they assessed and adapted.

One of the most admirable aspects of aviation is its relentless commitment to preparation. Whether it's a pilot's first flight or their 300th, checklists are followed. Procedures are drilled. Safety demonstrations, often ignored by frequent flyers, exist not for comfort but for survival.

Cronin and his team executed a rapid descent to a breathable altitude—a textbook maneuver they had drilled countless times. The co-pilot worked the radio, issuing a mayday call. The flight engineer scrambled to manage the aircraft's failing systems. The cabin crew, shaken but determined, calmed passengers and provided support. Everyone had a role. Everyone executed it.

With the aircraft still barely holding together, the pilots turned back toward Honolulu. Every movement was deliberate. Every checklist was followed. And after what must have felt like forever, the runway lights came into view. The crew landed the damaged 747 with precision. Of the 337 people originally on board, 328 survived.

Flight 811 is more than a tragic event; it's a powerful reminder that preparation saves lives. The crew didn't wing it. They didn't guess. They followed the steps, trusted their training, and relied on calm, collaborative execution.

Because when crisis strikes, improvisation rarely works. Clarity, preparation, and communication do.

Know Yourself, Know the Battle

Ideally, your daily life doesn't feel like a full-blown aviation emergency, but hearing about the structure, training, and checklist culture of aviation got me thinking about parenting and relationships, especially about how we prepare (or don't) for everyday chaos.

Take driving with kids, for example.

Few things test the limits of human patience like a car ride with young children.

You start with the best intentions: amazing plans, big adventures, and a solid strategy to get out the door. And, to your surprise, everything goes smoothly. The kids are dressed, the shoes are on the correct feet, and no one's thrown a tantrum about their snack choices. You even make it to the car without incident. Things are looking good.

But then, the second their little tushies hit those car seats, all chaos breaks loose. Suddenly, the backseat becomes a horror movie soundtrack—whining, shrieking, and bizarre demands raining down in surround sound: "Are we there yet?"

"I want my water!"

"NOT THAT SONG!"

"Snack! Snack! Snack!"

"Stop looking at me!"

"Are we there yet?" (Again. Two minutes later.)

"I didn't get my snack yet!"

"Are we there yet?"

You grip the steering wheel. You try deep breathing. You remind yourself they're just kids. But eventually, your nerves fray. You snap. Maybe it's a raised voice, a sarcastic comment, or the infamous hollow threat: "I'll turn this car around!"

But here's where it really gets messy.

You and your partner turn on each other.

It starts small:

"Can you deal with this?"

"Why didn't you pack the snacks?"

"Why didn't you take them to the bathroom before we left?"

Suddenly, you're in a full-blown argument about something completely unrelated. That thing they said last week? Now it's back. That unresolved tension from a few nights ago? Front and center. Meanwhile, the kids are still shouting in the back.

By the time you arrive, you're drained and disconnected. What was supposed to be a fun outing is now a minefield of tension. You glance at your partner and silently ask: how did we end up here?

These are the "wars" we fight, not against each other, but often beside each other, worn down by noise, fatigue, and unspoken needs.

One of my all-time favorite TV shows, *Modern Family*, nails this dynamic perfectly. While I've always loved Phil Dunphy (and his epic dad energy), it's Jay and Gloria's relationship that hits home for me for this topic. Their generational and cultural differences, plus Jay's second-time-around efforts to "get it right," make their dynamic rich with miscommunication and growth.

There's a moment I always come back to:

Jay walks in, leans in for a kiss, and Gloria recoils with obvious frustration.

Confused, Jay asks, "What's up? Are you mad at me?"

And Gloria delivers this iconic line:

"Did you do something to make me mad? If you did, I am mad. If you didn't, I am not."

It's hilarious. But it's also incredibly real.

That moment captures the emotional fog so many couples deal with. The guessing, the tiptoeing, the frustration of trying to connect while still trying to make sense of our reactions.

We end up fighting each other when we should be fighting *with* each other—on the same team, against the real issue. But that happens only when we pause long enough to ask the right questions and figure out what the real battle is.

There's More to Listening Than We Hear

In the article *Parables of Leadership*, author W. Chan tells a story that's left a lasting impression on me. Back in the third century, a young prince named T'ai was sent to study under the great master Pan Ku. As the future ruler of his people, the prince was expected to develop the wisdom and presence required to lead. But rather than start with strategy or governance, the master gave him a curious assignment:

"Spend a year alone in the Ming-Li Forest," he said. "Then return and describe all the sounds you hear."

After a year, the prince returned confident in his report. He listed birds singing, leaves rustling, bees buzzing, and the whisper of wind. He believed he had passed the test. But Master Pan Ku shook his head.

"Go back," he said. "Listen again. This time, tell me what more you can hear."

Frustrated but obedient, the prince returned to the forest. At first, it was the same symphony of familiar sounds. But as the days passed and he grew still, something shifted. He began to hear beyond the obvious. The faint sound of flowers blooming. The quiet warmth of the sun on the earth. Grass sipping morning dew. When he returned and shared his discovery, the master smiled.

"To hear the unheard," he said, "is the skill of a great ruler. Only when you learn to listen to what is not spoken—the fears, the pain, the needs hidden in silence—can you truly connect and lead others."[1]

This lesson wasn't just for a king. It's a lesson for every one of us trying to navigate relationships, especially when things feel tense or distant.

Most of us think we're good listeners. But if we're honest, many of us spend more time reacting than understanding. We're just waiting for our turn to talk. We react. We explain. We defend. Rarely do we pause long enough to wonder: *what is my partner really trying to say?*

Listening deeply, the kind of listening the prince had to learn, means paying attention not just to the words but to the emotions hiding beneath them. When your partner says, "You never help around the house," it's not really about the dishes. It might be about feeling unsupported or unimportant. When they say, "You're always on your phone," it's not about the screen; it's about feeling disconnected and unseen.

We hear the "rustling leaves" of our partner's complaints but fail to notice the "flowers blooming" in their silence, the deeper fears or frustrations they don't know how to express.

Listening at this level is hard because it requires vulnerability. It means sitting with discomfort. It means asking yourself tough questions: *What if they're lonelier than I realized? What if I missed something important? What if I've stopped showing up in ways that matter most?*

It's easier to argue about the surface issues of money, time, in-laws, or chores than to confront what's really going on: disconnection, hurt, fear, or longing.

We often mistake the sound of a slammed door for anger when it's really a cry to be noticed. We interpret silence as disinterest when it's really a fear of saying the wrong thing.

But when we start to listen differently, the whole dynamic changes.

You don't need to disappear into a forest for a year to become a better listener. You just need to shift your focus.

With the right tools, you'll be better equipped to handle whatever parenting challenges come your way, whether it's navigating the complexities of bedtime routines or figuring out who gets the last cup of coffee in the morning. And remember, love may be the foundation of your relationship, but how you listen during the wars is what determines if that foundation holds.

Fighting Happens, but Not Conflict

Disagreements are a regular part of any relationship, especially when you're raising kids together. You're two unique individuals with your own backgrounds, experiences, and state of mind, so it's only natural that you won't see eye to eye on everything.

I remember when I first started working with couples, I met a couple who came to therapy due to never having an argument and feeling like aliens among their family and friends. When I meet couples who aren't arguing, I get curious. Are they really that harmonious, or are they avoiding honesty? Are they being polite—or disconnected?

A few months ago, I was working with a client who was having a hard time expressing himself honestly. His fear? That being honest would trigger his partner, and things would spiral. I could empathize. Vulnerability feels risky. But I reminded him of something essential:

"Without expression, there is no awareness."

It sounds so simple and easy, but the expression part can be one of the biggest challenges of our relationships.

In the wise words of Brené Brown, "Clear is kind." Being open and expressive about your feelings isn't selfish; it's a gift to everyone involved because it clears up the mystery and builds connection. So, it might cause an argument or ruffle feathers for the short term, but if you never say anything, it will never get fixed; it ensures the issue stays unresolved, invisible, and festering.

The goal in a relationship isn't to avoid conflict altogether; it's to learn how to engage with it in a way that brings you closer. That requires showing up. Not floating on autopilot. Not pretending things are fine when they're not. And not burying resentment in the name of "keeping the peace."

Hard conversations are part of real love. And you don't need to have all the answers or like it; you just have to be willing to stay in the room when it gets tough. Robert Frost said, "The only way out is through." That's not just a poetic line; it's the map for growth.

Especially in parenting, conflict is often fueled by more than the moment itself. Maybe you're running on no sleep. Maybe the baby just threw up on your last clean shirt. Maybe you haven't had a real conversation with your partner in days. Suddenly, a tiny disagreement, like whether it's time to switch from bottles to sippy cups, morphs into a blowout over who's doing more, giving more, or carrying more mental load.

But here's what we forget in those moments: you're not opponents; you're a team.

Parenting stress makes it easy to forget that. So before you let a disagreement spiral into a battle, pause. Breathe. Remind yourself, we're on the same side.

That doesn't mean you won't fight. You will. But how you fight and how you recover is what makes all the difference.

The rest of this chapter will give you tools to manage those moments: to de-escalate, communicate clearly, and rebuild connection even when you're in the middle of the mess. Because love is the foundation, but communication is the blueprint for how you build and rebuild, again and again.

I Hear You

When you start hearing someone, something magical happens. When someone feels genuinely heard, a shift begins. They soften. They feel seen. They feel safe. And when people feel safe, they let their guard down.

Instead of yelling, they share. Instead of retreating, they open up.

This is where conflict begins to de-escalate. The arguments that used to spiral out of control start to slow down. You move past surface-level issues and start addressing the real roots of disconnection. Deep listening won't magically resolve every disagreement, but it will build understanding, and understanding is the foundation of trust, emotional safety, and love.

You start picking up on what your partner isn't saying. You notice when they're withdrawing before it erupts into a fight. You sense when they're overwhelmed before they can even name it. You learn to meet their needs not because they demanded it, but because you've become attuned.

That's not just a skill. It's a gift.

Listening this deeply is how we express love in the moments that matter most. It's how we say, "I see you. I hear you. I care about what you're going through, even when you're not saying it out loud."

As one of my favorite authors on love, Erich Fromm puts it:

"Love is an activity, not a passive affect; it is a 'standing in,' not a 'falling for.' In the most general way, the active character of love can be described by stating that love is primarily giving, not receiving."[2]

Love isn't just a feeling you fall into; it's something you *do*. It's an ongoing practice. A verb. A conscious effort. And the moment we stop working at it, the moment we start going silent or passive, that's when love begins to erode.

I once worked with a couple who came to therapy because they had stopped talking altogether. Conflict had worn them down. Arguments had turned into silence. They weren't fighting anymore, but they weren't connecting either. They were just passing each other in the hallway, heads down, emotionally checked out.

And when both partners stop trying, stop reaching, stop listening, that's when the real danger sets in.

So yes, love takes effort. Listening takes courage. And emotional presence requires practice. But these are the daily acts that say "I'm still here. I still care. I still choose you."

Standstill Traffic

Author Amanda Ripley wrote, "High conflict isn't always violent but is extremely flammable."[3] So how can we bring down the flames and truly connect during times of passion and fire within our relationships that feel too hot to handle?

According to relationship experts, Drs. John and Julie Gottman, there are three primary types of arguments couples experience:

- Solvable arguments (31%).
- Perpetual arguments (69%).
- And within that 69%, 16% become gridlock conflicts.

Solvable arguments are just what they sound like: issues that can be worked through with effort, communication, and compromise. There may be discomfort, but there's also a clear path forward.

Perpetual arguments are the repeat offenders. These are the issues that show up again and again, often tied to personality differences or deep values. They don't go away, but couples can learn to manage them with emotional intelligence and solid skills.

Then there are the *gridlock arguments*. Imagine rush hour in New York City or Los Angeles. No one is moving. Horns are blaring.

Everyone's frustrated. That's gridlock. These arguments feel impossible to escape. They're the emotionally charged, deeply rooted issues that loop endlessly with no progress. You get pulled into the same pain, frustration, and hopelessness every time.

Gridlocks make up only a small fraction of all conflicts, but they can pull us in the deepest. And if we're not careful, they can begin to define the relationship.

Activity: When There's Gridlock, Be the Traffic Helicopter

Whenever you are driving in traffic, everything seems to bother you, time moves slowly, and the world and everything in it sucks.

Now imagine you're not in the traffic; you're above it.

Think of yourself as the traffic helicopter flying overhead. You're not stuck; you're observing. You can see the cause of the jam: an accident, a lane closure, a bottleneck. You see the bigger picture.

Try applying that same principle in a gridlock argument:

- *Pause and rise above. When emotions escalate, pause. Imagine rising above the conflict like a helicopter viewing the whole scene.*
- *Observe, don't judge. Talk about what you see—patterns, stuck points, unmet needs without blame. "It looks like we're both feeling unheard," or "From above, I see us repeating the same cycle."*
- *Take turns. Let each partner share their "helicopter view" of the conflict without interruption or defensiveness.*
- *Stay curious. Approach it like a news crew analyzing a situation, not enemies in battle.*

This perspective creates emotional space. Instead of reacting from within the chaos, you're stepping outside it together. And that's often where healing begins.

Let Your Guard Down

Before we move forward, I want to pause and highlight something essential:

The goal of an argument isn't to win. It's not to be the loudest or to "get your point across."

The goal of an argument is to reach a deeper level of understanding.

In an ideal world, we'd approach every conflict with patience and grace—sitting down, making eye contact, speaking calmly. But in real life? We're tired. We're overwhelmed. We're emotionally tapped out. And sometimes, words come out sideways.

Deep down, we know better. The real work isn't about being perfect communicators. It's about using those human moments to gain insight, understand each other a little more, and keep growing closer, even when it's hard.

Many couples therapists use the phrase "the rainbow after the storm" as a symbol of repair. I get it. But here's the thing: not every storm ends with a rainbow. Sometimes, the clouds simply part a little. The sky gets less heavy. A sliver of light breaks through. That might not be magical, but it's real. And real is what we're after. Don't expect that just because you've talked it out and the weight feels lifted, everything is now sunshine and daisies. The work continues but now, you're walking through it together. There's a classic parable by philosopher Arthur Schopenhauer called *The Porcupine Dilemma.*

> On a cold winter's day, a number of porcupines huddled together for warmth, desperate to escape the bitter chill. But as they get closer to each other, they prick each other with their sharp quills and are forced to pull away. This cycle continues, drawing together for warmth, retreating from pain, until they discover a delicate balance: a distance where they are close enough to share warmth but far enough to avoid hurting one another. It's not perfect; the warmth is less than ideal, and the quills still sting and poke them from time to time. But it's tolerable, and that will be enough to survive.[4]

Relationships are like that.

We crave closeness, but closeness isn't always comfortable.

The more intimate the relationship, the more likely we are to bump into each other's sharp edges:

- The forgotten socks
- The missed texts
- The differing values
- The misunderstood tone
- The triggers and traumas we didn't even realize we carried

The challenge is finding that "moderate distance," the sweet spot where we can stay connected without causing unnecessary harm. It's a tricky balance, and sometimes we swing too far in one direction, clinging too tightly, or too far in the other, isolating ourselves in the name of self-preservation.

What Schopenhauer's porcupines teach us is that perfect harmony doesn't exist. Relationships are a balance, full of warmth and wounds, connection and conflict. The goal isn't to avoid pain altogether but to find a rhythm where the connection is worth the occasional prick. It's about learning when to lean in for warmth and when to step back to protect each other's boundaries.

When I work with individuals, especially those dating, I often use the metaphor of armor. We wear it to protect ourselves—from pain, from rejection, from past wounds. And while that armor keeps us safe, it also keeps people out. You can't build closeness from behind a wall.

Here's the hard truth:

You cannot crave connection while refusing vulnerability.

Letting your guard down is terrifying. But it's the only path to intimacy that matters. You can't fall in love while holding a shield.

The Michelangelo Effect

The last concept about how we deal with others before we get into the nitty-gritty of arguments and conflicts is the *Michelangelo Effect*.[5] This is the tendency many of us have (especially in early relationships) to see our partner not as they are but as a project—someone to sculpt into our version of "ideal." It's the voice in your head that says:

- "When we get engaged, they'll change."
- "After we get married, I'll work on that part of them."
- "Once we have kids, they'll step up."
- "When we get closer to making this official I'll make sure she acts, thinks, or behaves like X,Y,Z."

I heard it from friends when I was dating. I hear it from clients every week.

Here's my advice, plain and simple:

Stop dating and marrying potential.

Marry who you see today.

Yes, we all grow. Yes, people change. But love isn't about who someone *might* become—it's about who they are right now. If you're building your relationship on the foundation of "I'll fix them later," you're setting yourself up for frustration, resentment, and endless arguments with a ghost version of your partner that never existed.

That doesn't mean you shouldn't have standards or goals. But communicate them openly, early, and often. Share your hopes and values. Let your partner decide if that aligns with who they are and what they want. Don't bottle it up and then explode because they're not living up to a fantasy you never verbalized or something you saw on reality TV, Instagram, or your favorite rom-com.

And for the love of all things holy, stop expecting your partner to be Ryan Gosling from *The Notebook*. This is real life. They're not scripted. They leave dishes in the sink. They forget what you said two days ago. They probably don't even know how to do that "passionate rain kiss" thing. But they show up. They try. They love you. And that's what matters.

Your job as a partner is to love and appreciate your person for who they are today and what they bring to your life in the here and now. We can't predict or plan what your life and relationship will be like in 1–10 years, so how can you expect to know all the greatness your partner will become or the struggles you will go through?

You can't know, so live in these moments with the person you have in front of you today.

Love isn't about perfection. It's about presence.

It's about choosing each other, again and again even with the quirks, the disagreements, the socks on the floor.

Your job isn't to mold your partner into your ideal.

Your job is to love them for who they are today.

Because that's the only version of them you truly have.

Five Basic Myths About Conflict

Myth #1

Fighting = Divorce.

Truth

When I was first married, my mom and dad were always and still are an amazing source for relationship advice and experience. So after my first big argument with my wife, I turned to them to chat and process what happened. My mom said when my parents were first married and they got into their first argument, she began to cry intensely, not because of the argument but because she thought she and my father were getting divorced.

She never saw her parents argue and thought only problematic couples argued.

Every couple argues! Not all resolve, repair, and reset well, but that's for later.

You aren't having a problem in a relationship because you are arguing, you are just two humans trying to live their lives as one. . .you will butt heads.

What's important is the balance of arguments to neutral/calm/ happy moments and interactions. From the research,[6] it's a 5-to-1 ratio called the *magic ratio*. The five positive interactions can be anything from smiling at each other to date night to sex. It is something that brings closeness and love. When working with clients, I aim for a 70–30 ratio, with an ideal of 80–20. However, there will be months and years that lower the ratio.

Something I say to clients often who are in a state of arguing is, "At least you are communicating. It's not the best way to communicate, but you could be hating on each other so much that you stop talking entirely."

Myth #2

There are winners and losers.

Truth

If your goal in an argument is to win, you've already lost something much more important: connection.

Relationships aren't about keeping score. There's no scoreboard for who changed more diapers, who said sorry first, or who's more "right" about the laundry. But when we're exhausted, frustrated, and emotionally fried, it's easy to fall into that trap. Suddenly, every disagreement turns into a tally sheet. "I got up with the baby three nights in a row." "You didn't even load the dishwasher." Sound familiar?

I've seen this play out in the therapy room countless times. One couple came in ready for battle, both with mental spreadsheets of who did what and when. The wife felt like she was doing everything (and she had a list with her to read off), and the husband felt like no matter what he did, it wasn't enough. They weren't talking to each other; they were defending themselves, hoping the person would see them and appreciate all their hard work. The issue wasn't really about dishes or bedtime routines. It was about both of them feeling unseen and underappreciated, stuck in a loop of proving their worth instead of finding understanding.

And I've been guilty of it myself. I can remember a rough fight with my wife where I walked away feeling like I "won."

I made my point. I stood my ground. But when I saw her later, quiet and hurt on the couch, it hit me: I hadn't won anything that mattered. I'd bulldozed my way through the argument and left her emotionally alone. That kind of "victory" doesn't bring closeness. It builds walls.

The second we turn our relationship into a competition, we stop being teammates. We lose the "us" in all the noise of "me versus you." And that's not just damaging, it's lonely.

So what's the alternative? Shift your mindset from winning to understanding. Ask yourself, "Do I want to be right, or do I want us to be okay?" If you lead with curiosity instead of defensiveness, and prioritize connection over ego, you'll be surprised by how much less fighting there is and how much more healing happens.

Because in the end, love isn't about who scores more points. It's about showing up for each other, especially when it's hard, and remembering that you're on the same damn team.

Myth #3

Logic is better for arguments.

Truth

Logic has its place, but connection isn't built on bullet points or airtight arguments. Facts might win debates, but they don't heal hurt feelings.

I see this all the time with couples. One partner leans hard on logic during conflict, thinking, *If I can explain it clearly enough, this will all make sense and go away.* It's not usually malicious. Most of the time, it comes from a place of wanting to keep things calm and avoid escalation. But what starts as "being reasonable" can land as cold, dismissive, or disconnected, especially when what the other person needs is warmth and emotional presence.

I had a client once say to me, "I don't get why she's still upset. I explained exactly why I was late and that it wasn't my fault." And you know what? He *was* right on paper. But that wasn't the point. But she didn't care about the logistics of traffic or the calendar. What she felt was forgotten. Unimportant. Not prioritized. And no amount of explanation could soothe that feeling. What she needed to hear was something like, "I'm sorry I made you feel like you didn't matter. That wasn't my intention." That emotional acknowledgment would have gone a lot further than justifying the delay. She needed to know that he saw her pain and that he cared. All his logic only made her feel more alone.

In another session, a man told me flat out, "I can't empathize with her; it's too much work. I need more logic and calm in my life." I understood his exhaustion, truly. Emotional waves can feel overwhelming. But that's the reality of being in a relationship: you're not partnering with a robot. You're building a life with another human being who comes with feelings, needs, and their history. Empathy isn't optional if connection is the goal.[7]

You're not in court; you're in a relationship. You're not trying to win a case, you're trying to care for someone's heart. And that requires tapping into the emotional side, especially when things feel hard. Logic can help when you're figuring out chores or planning a schedule. But when the argument is emotionally driven, dwelling on it keeps you disconnected. You might feel "clear-headed," but your partner feels alone.

So, the next time you're in a tense moment, try pausing to reflect. Instead, ask yourself, "What does my partner need to feel right now: safe, heard, seen?" Connection isn't built by being the smartest person in the room; it's built by being the most emotionally present one.

If you really want to connect, don't lead with logic; lead with love.

Myth #4

It's best to run away from negativity.

Truth

Sweeping it under the rug just builds a mountain. When I was a teenager, my main chore was to clean my room weekly. I hated cleaning my room. I liked everything where it was and didn't care if it was a mess, but it was a responsibility I had as someone who lived in the house.

So, I got smart about it. Well, I thought I did. I would take all the things I could and throw them into the bottom and top of my closet, shove stuff under the bed and in drawers. From my parents' perspective and the outside, it looked like I cleaned my room (I probably didn't fool my parents at all, especially when I cleaned the room in less than five minutes, but they didn't argue with me).

As Dr. David Burns in *Feel Good Therapy*[8] says with this *under-the-rug* way of dealing with things, we then lose control of how the information and things unsaid or shoved in places will be stored. When we hide it, we are at the whim of the unknown. Anything and everything can open that closet a little too far, and the mountain of unsaid, dirty laundry and mess comes flying out.

This is what people do when they don't want to rock the boat or cause issues in their relationship. They avoid and hide from negativity. But what happens is a buildup of resentment. You don't have to share everything, but you need to share something. Negative feelings aren't bad. They can be intimidating at times, so seek help to develop better tactics for constructively expressing them.

Myth #5

You have to have it all figured out before getting into a relationship.

Truth

If this were the case, no one would be in a relationship!

We are all a work in progress. What you need to know about yourself is enough to show who you are. If you don't know more, let the person you are with ask questions and be curious so you can learn about each other together.

There is a cute story from the "Old Country":

There was a small town that was built by the ocean. The mayor instructed his people that whenever they needed water, they must build a filtration system to make the water usable. This became a law of the land and way of life for many generations. It became a part of their daily lives and something that was never tested or questioned.

One day, there was a fire in town, and the fire department ran out of water, so they went to the ocean and began their filtration process, because the rule was, don't use the water unless it is filtered. By the time they were done, many houses had burned down.

The mayor came out of his office and called a town hall meeting. In the meeting, he yelled at the fire department and anyone else who could have helped and said: "If there is a fire and your world is burning, you use whatever resource you have to save your town and its people."

Jenna and Marcus had always prided themselves on having a "no screens during dinner" rule. From the time their son Milo could hold a spoon, dinners were sacred, time to connect, talk about their day, and avoid distractions. It worked well. . .until it didn't.

One night, after an impossibly long day, Marcus had back-to-back Zoom calls, Jenna had been juggling toddler tantrums and deadlines, and Milo had a full-on meltdown at daycare and they sat down to dinner, exhausted. Milo, very tired and overstimulated, pushed his plate away and screamed, "I hate broccoli!" followed by inconsolable sobs. Jenna tried to soothe him. Marcus tried bribing with dessert. Nothing worked.

Then Milo gasped between cries, "I just wanna watch Bluey." Jenna and Marcus locked eyes. The rule. No screens. It had been their anchor. Their way of protecting family connection. Their thing.

"We don't do that, buddy. It's dinner," Marcus said, gently but firmly.

Milo screamed louder, kicked the table, and crumpled into a mess of tears.

Finally, Jenna whispered, "Screw it," pulled out the iPad, and put on Bluey. Milo calmed instantly, munching his dinner while watching. The silence was. . .glorious.

Marcus looked deflated, almost ashamed. "Did we just give up?" Jenna smiled softly. "No. We adapted. Tonight was ridiculous, and we are doing the best we can; we are just trying to survive."

Another couple I worked with had a similar experience. Maya and Devin were in a rough patch. They'd been working on their marriage for months but hadn't made progress. So Maya decided to plan a romantic dinner, a home-cooked meal, candlelight, and no phones. A gesture to reset the tone.

But that day, work ran late. The baby spit up on her dress. Devin walked in frustrated from traffic and forgot the flowers she had hinted about. Halfway through burnt lasagna and a baby monitor that wouldn't stop buzzing, Maya broke down. "Why do I even try?" she muttered through tears.

Devin sat down across from her, took her hand, and said, "Because you care. And I see it, even when things don't go as planned. We're both tired. But I'm here. Can we just eat cereal on the couch together and call it a win?"

They did. And laughed. And cuddled up with Netflix, no expectations, just presence.

They used whatever they could and it's still good enough and usable, not perfect.

Same thing for us, we feel so often that we need to know every nook and cranny about ourselves to be the best version of ourselves for a relationship. We feel like we have to filter all the good and bad things and have it all figured out. Well, your relationship needs you now. Use what you have and learn to grow through it all. There will be more time, new situations in life, and things that will teach you more about yourselves than all the thinking and introspection in the world. Don't wait to be perfect. Be real, and grow from there.

What Is the Focus?

According to Charles Duhigg in his outstanding book *Supercommunicators*,[9] he says there are three main things to focus on while arguing or in a heightened state of conflict:

- Yourself
- Your environment
- The conflict's boundaries

Let's walk through each of these because when arguments get loud or emotions run high, having a mental map makes all the difference.

Yourself

This one's first for a reason. You can't navigate conflict well if you don't know what's going on inside you.

"Yourself" refers to your internal state: your emotional regulation, mindset, and self-awareness in the heat of the moment. Have you created enough space to actually *be* in this conversation? Or are you coming in already flooded?

I know I struggle with getting overwhelmed, what therapists call *emotional flooding*. It's when emotions, thoughts, and sensations rush in all at once and hijack your system. You feel trapped, dysregulated, and completely unable to think clearly or respond with intention.

As someone with ADHD, I've always been extra sensitive to criticism. It doesn't just feel like feedback; it hits like failure. It's as if I'm not being told I messed up but that *I am the mess-up*. Through years of therapy, I came up with a name for this feeling: Flash Mode (more on that in Chapter 8). It's when my brain goes into hyperdrive, my thoughts race, and I feel like everything is slipping through my fingers.

Naming it helped me slow down. It reminded me that I wasn't broken; I just needed a different path to regulation.

Maybe it's a long day absorbing other people's stress. Maybe it's your kids yelling, or something as random as a Tuesday funk. Whatever it is, the key is learning to recognize your internal signals before they explode outward.

Reacting without self-awareness? That's on you.

Responding with intention? That's growth.

So, if you struggle with getting flooded, the key to help with the struggle is to become more aware of your inner triggers and warning signs that you are a ticking time bomb about to be set off and you work hard to slow down tools to calm yourself just a little bit to handle the situation better.

If you're prone to flooding or Flash Mode, here's what helps:

- **Recognize your cues:** Tight chest, racing thoughts, clenched jaw, urge to escape.
- **Take a break:** Stop and rest before you break down.
- **Name it out loud to your partner:** "I'm starting to feel overwhelmed. I want to do this conversation well—can we pause for a moment?"

That last one is powerful. Letting your partner into your headspace builds connection, not distance. It helps them understand where you are instead of assuming you're shutting down or lashing out.

As Professor Jon Kabbat-Zin wrote, "You can't stop the waves, but you can learn how to surf."[10] When you tell your partner what you are going through, you are letting your partner into your headspace and that can save a lot of disconnect and arguments.

Your Environment

This isn't just about physical space (we covered sacred spaces in Chapter 8). It's about the emotional climate of your day and what's going on *around* the argument.

What's the backdrop to this conflict?

- Have you been traveling nonstop?
- Did your kid throw a tantrum in target and you're still carrying the stress?
- Did something external—like a rough news cycle, social media doomscrolling, or a chaotic workweek—drain your bandwidth?

I saw this a lot during the pandemic and election cycles. Couples weren't just arguing about groceries or screen time; they were overwhelmed by uncertainty, grief, and nonstop digital noise. And that anxiety needed somewhere to go.

Knowing your emotional environment can save you from misinterpreting or escalating.

Ask yourself and each other:

- "What's really going on today?"
- "Is this about us, or is the world seeping in?"

Activity: Force Field

In every good sci-fi movie—from Star Wars *to* Star Trek—*there's a force field protecting the ship from external attacks. You can create something similar for your relationship.*

When life gets chaotic, kids are melting down, work is overwhelming, or the news cycle is triggering, build a shared "force field." This isn't about physical barriers (though your bedroom might be one!) but about establishing emotional boundaries and mutual understanding.

Here's how to create one:

- *Choose a space that feels like a refuge (bedroom, porch, car ride, etc.).*
- *Name the emotional needs: quiet, affection, no problem-solving, venting-only, etc.*

(continued)

(continued)

- *Agree on when to activate the force field—after school, before bed, post-family visit.*
- *Keep it flexible. Like an import/export list, this will evolve with your life phases.*

The goal isn't perfection. It's protection of your connection, your peace, and your emotional safety as a couple.

The Conflict Boundaries

Arguments can feel like emotional avalanches. One minute you're talking about dishes, and the next, you're bringing up something from 2017 involving a forgotten birthday and your mother-in-law's side comment about your cooking. Why? Because once the gates of honesty swing open, it's tempting to dump every grievance you've been storing. This is what Drs. John and Julie Gottman call *kitchen sinking.*[11]

I call it the *list.*

Most of us have a mental list of big hurts, minor annoyances, and unresolved frustrations that we hold onto like ammo, just in case. When we feel cornered or criticized, we reach for it. Suddenly, the conversation takes a left turn. The original issue is gone, and now the spotlight is on your partner's flaws instead of the shared conflict.

So here's my advice: *throw the damn list out.*

This isn't money in the bank or saved-up vacation days. These are emotional landmines. Stockpiling them only builds resentment, mistrust, and fear. You say you love this person, but why are you keeping score like you're waiting to win a debate? If you're storing up grievances like a hunter in the bushes, you're preparing for war, not connection. Burn the list and stay here, in *this* moment.

As Ekhart Tolle put it beautifully, "Wherever you are, be there totally."[12]

That's the art of presence. And it's the antidote to kitchen sinking.

You might feel that if you don't get this idea in now or say it right now it'll be lost forever and the opportunity is gone, but you can always bring things up later; not everything has to be solved today. As the Gottmans say so beautifully, "Solve the moment, not the fight."[13]

Learning to prioritize the *now* over *everything* is a skill that can transform your communication, not just in romantic relationships but with your kids, friends, and co-workers, too.

I know how hard this can be, especially if, like me, you grew up struggling to hold your tongue. My ADHD brain used to scream at me during conversations:

"Say it now before it's gone!"

When I was doing that, I wasn't *listening*. I wasn't present. I was so busy prepping my next point that I missed the moment in front of me. It's selfish, honestly, assuming that every thought you have deserves the floor, even if it steamrolls your partner in the process.

So here's a simple, no-BS tool I give clients:

Carry a small notepad.

When your brain is screaming to interrupt or go off-topic, write the thought down. Make it clear to your partner that this isn't a scoreboard; it's your *interruption protector*. You're not taking notes to build a case. You're simply giving your brain a safe place to park the thought so you can stay grounded in the present.

It's like in therapy: a client sees the therapist scribble something and instantly thinks, *Oh no, did I say something wrong?* But most of the time, it's just the therapist jotting down a keyword or yes, doodling a little. (Sorry, therapists, for outing us.)

This tool does two things:

- It validates your thought—you don't have to ignore it.
- It buys you time—so you can decide later if it's even worth bringing up.

Because often, with space and perspective, you realize. . .it wasn't.

You Had Me at Hello

C.S. Lewis said, "You can't go back and change the beginning, but you can start where you are and change the ending."[14] And when it comes to conversations, especially the hard ones, that couldn't be more true.

According to powerful research by Drs. John and Julie Gottman, we have just *180 seconds*—that's three minutes—to change the direction and tone of a conversation. Three minutes might not sound like much, but in the heat of a tough moment, it's a lifetime. And it's enough time to shift everything. However, it takes a massive amount of awareness to shift the energy and momentum of the conversation. If you notice things escalating, you have the power to pause, breathe, and reset the emotional temperature. You don't need to fix the whole problem; you just need to steer the conversation in a better direction.

As a massive hockey fan, I am always enamored with the power of how small moments can change the momentum of a game. Announcers will say, "The ice is tilting," referring to a shift in energy. A well-timed penalty kill or a short, powerful 30-second shift can light a fire under a team and change the course of the entire game.

We have the ability and strength to change the way our conversations go.

We can shift the "ice" in our conversations, too. That shift depends on three things:

- The *energy* you bring
- The *environment* you're in
- The *boundaries* you've set around the conversation

And let's not underestimate the importance of *how* you start. A gentle, respectful open can go a long way toward building connection, safety, and openness. Like I mentioned in Chapter 8, try simple entry points like these:

- "Do you have a moment to chat about something that's been on my mind?"
- "I've been feeling something lately and I'd love to talk about it—would now be a good time?"

These aren't magic spells, but they are meaningful cues. They give your partner a chance to step into the conversation willingly instead of feeling ambushed. That little bit of emotional buy-in at the start can change everything.

So the next time you feel the energy shifting or sense a conflict brewing, remember:

You've got three minutes. Use them wisely.

Gameplan

When conflict arises, we tend to fall into a few predictable traps that, while understandable, can do serious damage to the relationship if left unchecked. Let's walk through those patterns and build a better game plan.

Getting Space

Needing space isn't the problem. It's how we take it that matters.

Sometimes you're overwhelmed, overstimulated, or just too heated to keep talking. So, what happens? One person storms off, slams a door, or disappears without a word. The other is left feeling abandoned, panicked, or furious.

Let's shift this dynamic with a simple, three-step framework:

If you're the one leaving:

1. **Confirmation + Comfort:**
   "Hey babe, I love you and I want to keep talking, but I need a few minutes to cool off."
2. **Time Frame:**
   "Give me 10–20 minutes to reset."
3. **Return:**
   "When I get back, I'd like to keep talking about [insert topic]."

If you're the one staying:

Let them go. Don't chase, don't guilt, don't push. Space isn't rejection; it's regulation. Giving your partner breathing room shows trust, and that trust builds safety.

Taking space is healthy. Storming off without context? That's just an adult tantrum in disguise.

When Things Cross the Line

Sometimes, we cross a line, say something sharp, cutting, or dismissive, and the air instantly changes. The other person shuts down, and the conversation derails.

Here's a (slightly playful but effective) tactic I use with clients:

Throw the flag.

Yep, grab a dishtowel, this is your relationship's penalty flag. If your partner says something that stings deep, toss the towel in the air. That's your signal: something hurt. Now pause. Name it. Talk it through.

Important: This isn't about shaming or stopping the conversation—it's about protecting the connection. Once you've addressed the wound, pick the towel back up and keep going.

Don't let those moments linger in silence. Silence grows resentment. Express. Repair. Move on.

Rehash

A lot of people are terrified to do this in their relationships because the response on the other end is:

- Didn't we resolve this?
- Why are you still holding on to this?
- Oh my goodness, get over it already.

Revisiting a past issue can trigger defensiveness or shame, especially if it seems "resolved." But just because something is settled on the outside doesn't mean it's settled on the inside.

In my relationship, and with many clients, we call this the Rumpus Moment. Why? Because *rumpus* is my favorite word. It means to dance, release the tension, and let it out. It's not about reigniting old fights; it's about creating space to speak feelings that still linger.

Guidelines for a Rumpus Moment:

- **Approach with gentleness:** If your partner brings something up again, respond with kindness, not condescension.
- **Use this phrasing structure:**
  Topic → Feeling → Clarifying Question

Here are some examples of how to use the formula:

a. "When we disagreed about how to handle Max's tantrum, I felt like you didn't have my back. Did I come off too strong or something?"
b. "Earlier, when I was talking and you were on your phone, I felt ignored. Were you just distracted?"
c. "When we started arguing in front of your family, I felt embarrassed and a little exposed. Was that how you were feeling too, or was I reading it differently?"
d. "Lately, I've felt something is off between us, like we've been disconnected. I've been wondering if something is up?"

Deconstructive Statements	Constructive Statement
"I hate it when you yell at me in the bouncy house."	"When we were yelling at each other in the bouncy house, I felt embarrassed and overwhelmed. Is that what you were feeling too?"
"You never listen to me."	"I feel unheard when I'm sharing something important and you look away. Were you distracted or feeling something else at that moment?"
"You're so selfish when we're with your family."	"When we're with your family, I sometimes feel left out. I'm wondering if you noticed that too or if you felt something different?"
"You always make everything about you."	"Sometimes I feel like my needs get overlooked. Can we talk about how to make space for both of us?"
"You don't care how I feel."	"It felt lonely when I was upset and you didn't respond. I'm trying to understand what was going on for you. Was it hard to know how to help me?"

How to Respond:

- Validate their feeling.
- Clarify your intention.
- Make a repair plan moving forward.

Here are some example responses (matching the previous situation):

a. "That's fair, and I see what you mean. I do trust you. I wasn't trying to step on your toes; I just panicked. Maybe next time we can pause and check in before jumping in?"

b. "I get why that bugged you. I would feel that way too. I wasn't trying to dismiss you; I just zoned out. I'll try to make an effort to put my phone down when we're having a real conversation."

c. "Yeah, that wasn't great. I didn't mean to put you in that spot; I got lost in the moment. Let's keep stuff like that between us next time."

d. "I hear you. It's not about you; I've just been in a weird head-space, but I just didn't know how to bring it up. Let's find some time this week, just the two of us."

When we allow for rehashing without judgment, we stop pain from festering. We give our partner the gift of being heard, even if it's the second time around.

Not too long ago, I had a small, seemingly mundane interaction with my wife that caught me off guard:

Me: "Hi babe, can I soak this dish for a bit? The mess is getting a bit crusty, and I need to clear the sink. Is that okay?"

Wife: "Wait, why do you need to clear the sink? I need the sink the way it is so I can put things in there throughout the day, and the dishwasher is full!"

This interaction confused me so much, I thought I was asking something simple, more of a logistical conversation, and it felt like I touched a nerve.

About an hour or so later, my wife came over and called *Rumpus*.

She explained that my comment triggered a feeling of shame. She felt like I was pointing out a mess she made and it hit a nerve. She realized it wasn't my intention, but she needed me to know why it hurt.

We talked. We understood. We moved on.

Had we not made space for that Rumpus, who knows what would've bubbled up later? A misread moment could've turned into a multiday disconnect. But instead, it became a quick repair, a deepening of trust, and a reminder that even the smallest exchanges carry meaning.

Repair and Reset

Now that we have gone through some of the main key points of how to handle conflict, what causes conflict, and how to get through it smarter, let's dive into the last part, which is how to heal and move forward.

A common misconception is that repair means everything goes back to normal, like nothing happened. We aren't fruit flies that have the shortest memory and recall!

Arguments, especially the big, emotional ones, leave a mark. They take energy. They linger. So if we want to move forward together, we have to be intentional about how we heal.

Here are a few key pieces to true repair that lasts:

Apologize + Debrief   Once the dust has settled and emotions have cooled, that's your moment *not to pretend it never happened* but to step into it with more clarity and care.

Start with an honest apology. Not a perfect one, just a *real* one.

Your apology should reflect accountability. Maybe you raised your voice, dismissed their feelings, shut down, or made it about you when it wasn't. Whatever your role was, own it because most arguments aren't one-sided. We all play a role, even if it's not equal.

If you're waiting for a perfectly worded apology with flawless "I" statements and a step-by-step breakdown of exactly what they did wrong, when, and how, you're setting yourself up for disappointment. Your partner isn't a robot programmed for emotional perfection. They're human just like you. They may not say precisely what you *want* to hear. But if they're making an effort, if they're being honest and vulnerable, don't get stuck nitpicking the delivery. Focus on the heart behind it.

Genuine trumps polished every time.

Once the air feels a little clearer, that's when you can debrief. Talk about what triggered each of you, what escalated the argument, and how you can support one another better next time.

When it comes to balancing positive and negative interactions in a relationship, a good goal is to aim for about 70% to 80%

positive moments and no more than 20% to 30% negative ones. That doesn't mean being perfect; it means intentionally leaning toward a healthier balance, one repair at a time.

A question I get asked is:

> What if the dust has settled and I am not in the mood, too drained, and not interested in apologizing and the other person is?

Simple. Let them go first.

You don't have to match their emotional readiness if you're not there yet. Instead, receive the gesture with grace and honesty:

> "Thank you for saying that. I appreciate it and I feel seen by your apology. I'm still processing and need a little more time to fully own my part, but I promise I'll come back to it when I can."

That level of self-awareness matters. And while your partner may not love that answer in the moment; it's still a respectful, honest response. When your apology does come, it will be from a place of truth, not obligation. And that makes all the difference.

The whole point of repair isn't to erase the argument; it's to *learn* from it. It's a doorway to deeper understanding, more authentic intimacy, and a relationship where both of you feel safe enough to come back to the table, even after things get messy.

So take the time. Take the space. But don't miss the opportunity.

This is where a real connection is forged.

Reset Button

In my marriage, I've started using a simple tactic to shift the energy after a tough moment, one that blends humor, lightness, and love. It works only when the timing is right and we're both in agreement, but when it lands, it's powerful.

We call it the *reset button*.

For us, it's something playful: we each boop or gently squeeze the other's nose. That's it. It sounds silly, but it signals something meaningful: "I'm here. I still love you. Let's reset."

I use this with my kids, too. After big emotions, meltdowns, or moments when I've lost my cool, a little nose boop becomes our shared language of repair. It doesn't erase what happened. It just means we're ready to move forward together.

That said, timing matters.

I wouldn't recommend cracking a dad joke or trying to lighten the mood too quickly. Humor that feels dismissive can make your partner feel like you're minimizing the argument or their feelings. So if you're going to bring levity into the mix, make sure it's loving, not deflective. Reconnection doesn't mean pretending everything's perfect; it just means you're both ready to come back to each other.

Allow Space

Everyone processes differently. Some people need 10 minutes. Others need an hour or more. And that's okay. What matters is that we don't rush our partner—or ourselves—back to "normal."

I struggle with this. I'm quick to get fired up and just as quick to move on, ready to reset like nothing ever happened. But my wife sometimes needs more time. And honoring that difference has taken real effort.

If you're someone who needs space, try communicating it clearly so your partner doesn't feel shut out:

- "I'm okay, I just need a little more time to feel grounded again."
- "Thank you for talking through that with me. I'm still coming down emotionally—just need a bit more time to fully feel like myself."

That's how you make space feel safe rather than distant.

Reconnect

Now comes the reconnection. And let's get one thing clear: *recon-nection is not the same as make-up sex.*

Yes, intense emotions can lead to heightened passion, but when sex becomes the primary (or only) way to feel close again, it can set up a dangerous dynamic. I've worked with many couples who rely on conflict to fuel their intimacy. They crave the fire but don't know how to be close in the calm. That creates a cycle of chaos not connection.

True reconnection is about restoring your sense of "us." For some couples, that might be a hug, a kiss, or a quiet moment snuggled on the couch. For others, it's a date night, a shared laugh, or just holding hands while watching your favorite show. It doesn't have to be dramatic; it just has to be intentional.

It's the signal that says: *We're good. We're back on the same team.*

No one is born naturally great at communication or relationships. Not you, not your partner, not me.

These aren't talents, they're skills.

Learned. Practiced. Screwed up. Tweaked. Relearned.

It's a muscle we have to keep flexing, especially when life throws tantrums in the backseat, gridlocked arguments at dinner, and emotional landmines in the living room. The good news? That means no one is behind. You're not failing; you're learning. You're human.

If you take one thing away from this chapter, let it be this: conflict isn't a sign your relationship is broken. Avoiding it, numbing through it, or weaponizing it is where the danger lies. Arguments aren't the enemy. Silence, disconnection, and unresolved hurt are. The goal isn't to never fight; it's to fight fair, to recover well, and to use every moment as an invitation to grow closer rather than drift apart.

Because love isn't a destination, and it's not a highlight reel. It's a daily, imperfect effort. It's showing up, screwing up, repairing, and choosing each other again anyway. So don't waste time waiting to be "ready" or "perfect." Use what you have, where you are. And start shaping something real.

If you've made it this far, take a deep breath; you've just walked through the bumpy and meaningful terrain of conflict, communication, and repair.

This chapter wasn't about avoiding fights; it was about fighting smarter. About owning your stuff, offering grace, and building the kind of emotional safety that lets both people feel seen, heard, and chosen. Again and again.

Communication is only part of the equation. Because once the dust settles and the makeup hugs are exchanged, life continues. And that life? It's demanding, especially when you're raising tiny humans together.

Parenting doesn't just test your patience; it tests your partnership.

It's one thing to handle a disagreement about laundry or logistics. It's another to stand shoulder-to-shoulder during sleep regressions, toddler meltdowns, and the never-ending game of "Whose turn is it?" That's where the next chapter begins.

Because once the communication tools are in place, the next challenge is using them *together*. It's about shifting from "me versus you" to "us versus the chaos." It's about building a united front, not just in conflict, but in the day-to-day moments of parenting that ask us to be teammates, not opponents.

So as we move forward, let's talk about what it means to be on the same team, even when life makes it hard to remember that you are.

Notes

1. W. Chan Kim, and Renée Mauborgne, "Parables of Leadership," *Harvard Business Review* 70, no. 4 (1992): 123–128.
2. Erich Fromm, *The Art of Loving: The Centennial Edition* (A&C Black, 2000).
3. Amanda Ripley, *High Conflict: Why We Get Trapped and How We Get Out* (Simon and Schuster, 2022).
4. Arthur Schopenhauer, *Parerga and Paralipomena: Short Philosophical Essays*. Translated by R. J. (Cambridge University Press, 2000).
5. Caryl E. Rusbult et al., "The Michelangelo Phenomenon," *Current Directions in Psychological Science* 18, no. 6 (2009): 305–309.
6. John M. Gottman, and Nan Silver, *The Seven Principles for Making Marriage Work: A Practical Guide from the Country's Foremost Relationship Expert* (Harmony Books, 1999).
7. Empathy can be very hard for most people. To put yourself in someone else's mindset and be able to feel their way of perceiving the world is sometimes impossible. Try for sympathy, which means "I see you are struggling or have a feeling, and I care about you, so I care that you have feelings, and those matter to me."

8. David D. Burns, *Feeling Good*, 2nd ed. (Harper, 2000).

9. Charles Duhigg, *Supercommunicators* (Random House Publishing Group, 2025).

10. Jon Kabat-Zinn, *Wherever You Go, There You Are: Mindfulness Meditation in Everyday Life* (Hachette UK, 2023).

11. John Schwartz Gottman, and Julie Schwartz Gottman, *Fight Right: How Successful Couples Turn Conflict into Connection* (Random House, 2024).

12. Eckhart Tolle, *The Power of Now: A Guide to Spiritual Enlightenment* (New World Library, 2010).

13. Gottman and Gottman, *Fight Right*.

14. Attributed to C.S. Lewis.

10

Us vs. Them

"I can do things you cannot, you can do things I cannot; together we can do great things."

—Mother Teresa

TEAMWORK IS THE backbone of any successful partnership, whether in sports, business, or parenting. At home, it's what keeps the daily chaos from completely taking over. Even when life throws you a hectic and chaotic situation, it's the strength of your collaboration that keeps the family afloat.

Whether it's managing a never-ending bedtime routine, juggling chores, or simply making sure your kids leave the house in weather-appropriate clothes and matching socks, staying connected and cooperative with your partner is essential.

Even in the best of partnerships, there will be moments when your needs don't quite line up. And that's okay. What matters is how you navigate those moments with empathy and flexibility, recognizing that each partner's needs may carry different weight at different times.

I am a massive fan of comedy. Whether it's a stand-up special, a well-timed sketch, or a ridiculous YouTube clip, humor gives me a way to process life's intensity—especially in my work as a therapist. It offers perspective, invites levity, and helps me find light in the mess.

A few years ago, there was a fantastic bit by Chris Rock[1] about the power of being the tambourine player. In the bit, he talks about how, in a relationship, sometimes you get to be the lead singer belting out the big notes, and sometimes, you're in the back playing the tambourine. From the outside, the lead singer has it all and is rocking it. It might feel more glamorous to be center stage, but without the tambourine keeping the beat, the whole song can fall apart.

Parenting works the same. There are moments when one of you steps forward and takes charge: leading bedtime, handling the pediatrician calls, managing the logistics of a chaotic morning. And there are times when you're quietly supporting, doing the behind-the-scenes work that keeps the household humming (changing the diaper bag and loading the dishwasher). These roles are fluid. One moment you're rocking a fussy toddler to sleep (tambourine); the next, you're knee-deep in a potty-training crisis (lead vocals).

What matters most isn't who's doing what; it's how you move together. Supporting one another through those shifts is what defines the strength of the team. Sometimes, your needs will take a backseat so your partner can step up, and other times, they'll do the same for you. That's the rhythm of real partnership.

Imagine your partner walks through the door after an exhausting day at work. They're running on fumes and ask for just 15 minutes of quiet before jumping into the evening routine. That's your cue to pick up the tambourine—to keep things moving while they regroup. It's about giving them the space to decompress, knowing that your time to take the lead will come too, maybe tomorrow, when you've had a tough day and need to tap out for a bit.

This give-and-take is at the heart of what makes teamwork in parenting so powerful. It's not about keeping score or making sure everything is split exactly 50/50; it's about being attuned to each other's needs and finding a rhythm that works for your family. Just like in the bit, it's about knowing when to step forward and when to step back, when to let your partner take center stage, and when to play that supportive role. And sometimes, it's about recognizing that even the tambourine player deserves a standing ovation now and then.[i]

Support from the background isn't secondary; it's essential. Sometimes, being in the background means you're the one holding it all together, providing the foundation that allows your partner to shine. And that's no small deed. Whether it's managing the household logistics, keeping the kids entertained so your partner can finish that work deadline, or just being the one who always knows where the extra toilet paper is stashed, these are the moments that keep the family functioning. Just because these acts don't come with applause doesn't mean they aren't worthy of appreciation. In fact, they're often the most powerful demonstrations of love and commitment.

When you and your partner approach parenting with this kind of teamwork, you're not just making life easier; you're modeling something powerful for your kids. *They see that it's okay to need help sometimes, that it's essential to support the people you care about, and that every role, no matter how big or small, matters.* They don't just hear your words; they watch your behavior. They learn that relationships aren't about who does more or who's in charge; they're about collaboration, respect, and making sure everyone's needs are met, even if it's not all at the same time.

So when you find yourself playing the tambourine, holding the rhythm while your partner takes the lead, remember: you're not just filling in. You're maintaining harmony. And when it's your turn to step into the spotlight, trust that your partner will do the same for you.

---

[i] This concept of parenting and relationships being 50/50 is extremely wrong and unhealthy. Please look back at Chapter 2. We need to get out of the narrative that we both have to split everything down the middle. It isn't supposed to be fair or equal, life just needs to get done. For some days 100% is the energy you have to give and are you giving your all, not the actual amount.

This dynamic isn't always easy. In my therapy practice, I often see couples fall into a mindset of "me versus them," which can create such a cycle of resentment and comparison toward them for being the lead at this time. Remember, this is a momentary situation and not a forever thing. Stop treating your relationship like a competition. *If all you care about is who is winning or getting the spotlight, you're probably losing.*

Tip #1: Find Your Position

One of the most effective things you can do as a couple is take inventory of your strengths and limitations, not to judge or criticize, but to build a strategy. Sit down together and openly discuss what each of you does well and what areas may need support.

Think of it like building a championship team. The best coaches don't expect every player to master every skill. Instead, they create a roster where each person plays to their strengths and covers for one another's weaknesses. As Coach Mike Krzyzewski once said, "To me, teamwork is the beauty of our sport, where you have five acting as one. You become selfless." The same is true in parenting.

In my marriage, for example, my wife is phenomenal at managing logistics. She keeps track of the calendar, the little details, the moving parts that make up our family's daily life. It's a gift and sometimes a burden, but it's something she excels at. That doesn't mean I check out. It means I recognize that she's the captain of that domain, and I do everything I can to support, encourage, and lighten the load when I can.

On the other hand, I bring a lot of energy, humor, and flexibility into our home. I'm often the one goofing off with the kids, keeping things light, or playing host when we entertain. That doesn't mean my wife isn't fun; she is. But this is a role I naturally step into, and over time, it's become part of how we divide responsibilities.

The point isn't to stick each other in rigid roles; it's to communicate, adapt, and move fluidly as life requires. Knowing where each of you shines allows you to build trust, reduce friction, and operate from a place of mutual respect. It's not about doing everything equally. It's about showing up fully, together.

Chores + Life

One of the most common sources of tension in relationships is household labor—the endless dishes, the overflowing laundry, the mental checklist that never quite empties. But these tasks aren't just logistical; they're emotional. When one partner feels like they're carrying more than their share, it breeds frustration.

As a therapist, I've seen couples try to solve this with adult chore wheels. Personally? I'm not a fan. What I believe in more deeply is shared ownership. The home belongs to both partners. That means cleaning, cooking, organizing, and everything in between is not the job of one person; it's everyone's responsibility.

Rather than assigning tasks arbitrarily, I recommend a more thoughtful approach: talk about what you each enjoy, what you're good at, and what feels manageable. Use that to create a rhythm that works for both of you. But even when tasks are loosely divided, flexibility is key.

In my home, my usual tasks include taking out the garbage, cleaning the dog poop, and other heavy lifting duties around the house. My wife is usually in charge of packing lunches, doing dishes, and folding laundry. But that's not written in stone. If one of us is tired, overwhelmed, or busy, the other steps in. That's the unspoken agreement: *we show up for each other, not just the task list.*

There are a few essential truths here:

- **There is no perfect split:** What matters is that both people feel seen, valued, and supported.
- **Being tired is not a free pass:** Both of you are tired in different ways. Compassion matters more than comparison.
- **Not knowing how to do something is not an excuse:** If you don't know how to use the washing machine, ask. If you've never made the school lunches, learn. Being part of the team means building the skills to carry the weight.
- **Your upbringing isn't a fixed blueprint:** If you were raised in a household with traditional or unequal divisions of labor, you may need to challenge what you've internalized. Revisit the "Import/Export" exercise from earlier in this book to explore how expectations around home life were shaped and which ones you want to carry forward.

Shared labor is about respect. You're not doing chores to earn points. You're caring for your environment and each other. The sink full of dishes, the unfolded laundry, the bedtime routine—they're not just tasks. They're opportunities to support and invest in your partnership.

Parenting isn't glamorous. And when it comes to the day-to-day grind, diapers, vomit, bath time, and tantrums, it's easy to fall into default roles based on habit and upbringing. If you want to be respected as a partner, you have to show up for the whole experience. Not just the fun parts. Not just the parts you're comfortable with. *All of it.*

I remember a moment during the early days of the pandemic, when we were living with my parents. My daughter had a full-on poop explosion on herself, the couch, and my father. My dad, who had never changed a diaper in his life, panicked. He burst into the room where I was in session with a client and begged for backup. Diaper duty just wasn't something he ever saw as "his role."

But in today's world, that mindset no longer works. If you're in a parenting partnership, you don't get to opt out of the messy parts. Life doesn't always give you the option to wait for your partner. They might be out, sick, working, or simply burnt out. That's when you step up, take the reins, and keep the family moving forward.

Because parenting isn't about roles—it's about reliability. Can your partner count on you to handle the 3 a.m. wake-ups? To clean the throw-up? These aren't chores; they're challenges of commitment and demonstrations of love.

To soothe the toddler in the middle of a meltdown? If you want to be seen as an equal parent, you have to be present for the hard parts too.

Enemies No More

If you've ever traveled with young kids, you know it has the power to turn even the most laidback parents into tightly wound, irritable versions of themselves. A few years back, my wife and I discovered this firsthand. Every time we flew with our daughter, we inevitably ended up turning on each other due to the overwhelming stress that travel often brings. The intensity of managing bags, navigating airport security, handling tantrums, and dealing with delays, all while trying not to lose your sanity. Instead of supporting each other, we'd snap, argue over little things, and feel completely disconnected. It wasn't just frustrating; it hurt. It felt like we'd lost sight of something essential; *we were on the same side*. Eventually, we realized we had to approach these moments differently. Instead of just surviving them, we had to plan for them.

Before a trip, a big family event, or even a jam-packed weekend, we now take time to sit down and map it out. We talk through logistics, anticipate stress points, and, most importantly, remind each other that we're a team. A mentor once told me, "If you fail to plan, you plan to fail."[ii] That truth has stuck with me ever since.

Part of our planning includes safe words—playful but intentional signals we use when we feel ourselves starting to spiral. One of our favorites is "Sassafras." It's a nudge that says, "Hey, our attitude is slipping. Let's recalibrate." Another one is "Ginseng," our shorthand for: "We're in this together. Let's not lose sight of that." These words don't magically solve the situation. But they create a moment of pause, a shared language that helps us step out of the chaos and back into connection.

Sometimes we take it a step further. If things are really tense, one of us will initiate physical connection: a hand on the shoulder, a squeeze of the hand, or simply looking each other in the eyes. That grounding moment resets the energy and reaffirms our shared mission.

Stressful moments are inevitable. But how you show up for each other in them can either drive a wedge or deepen your bond. Choose the latter: connection over conflict, preparation over panic, and partnership over blame.

It's Not Your Job

Again and again, I see couples fall into the draining trap of believing it's their job to make their partner happy. Let me be clear: it's not. You are not responsible for anyone else's emotional state. You can influence it, support it, and create an environment where

---

[ii] Often attributed to Benjamin Franklin.

your partner feels seen and safe, but you are not the source of their happiness. And when you start believing that you are, it's a fast road to burnout, resentment, and disconnection.

Think of yourself as the sauce, not the main dish. You add flavor. You elevate the experience. But you are not the entirety of someone's emotional well-being. That's their job. Just like your emotional wellness is your responsibility.

The pressure to constantly monitor, manage, and "fix" your partner's mood will leave you feeling powerless and defeated. Why? Because no matter how hard you try, you can't control someone else's internal experience. And you're not supposed to.

The same truth applies to parenting. Your role as a parent isn't ensuring constant happiness; it's about creating an environment where all emotions are valid and welcome. When you push a "happy or nothing" narrative, you're unintentionally building a high-pressure environment that can linger for years. It sends the harmful message that emotions besides happiness aren't safe or acceptable, and that's a damaging message to carry into adulthood.

The antidote is permission. Permission to feel, express, and be human, without judgment or repair. So take the pressure off. Let go of the belief that your worth is tied to how happy you can keep everyone around you. Your role is to be present, grounded, and emotionally honest.

Let Them

In Chapter 6, I talked about a common dynamic where one parent, often the mother, accidentally sidelines the other. It usually comes from a place of care or concern: "Will they do it right? Will they pack the right snacks? Dress the baby appropriately? Say the right thing when the meltdown starts?"

If you want teamwork to thrive, you have to be willing to let your partner try, mistakes and all.

That doesn't mean abandoning them or watching from the sidelines with a smirk, waiting for them to get it wrong. It means giving them space to show up, figure it out, and grow into their role.

There's a difference between testing someone and challenging them. Testing sets someone up to fail; challenging offers them the opportunity to rise.

Letting go of control can feel risky, especially if you've spent a lot of time carrying the invisible weight of the household or parenting responsibilities. But part of true partnership is learning to trust each other's process, even if it looks different from yours.

That doesn't mean throwing your partner into the deep end without support. It means giving them room to take responsibility, develop their own rhythm, and gain confidence even if the diaper ends up backwards the first time.

When both partners are given the freedom to participate fully, even imperfectly, the relationship grows stronger. You each build self-trust, mutual respect, and shared ownership not just of tasks but of the emotional labor behind them.

You Can Ask for Help

There is this weird phenomenon of people thinking they need to finish what they started, even when it comes at the detriment of their own mental health and well-being.

Say it with me: asking for help is always okay!

It's a sign of strength, self-awareness, and respect for yourself, your partner, and your family.

You are not failing because your plan didn't work today. You are not a burden because you need a break. Asking for support communicates something powerful: "I trust you. I believe we're in this together."

I used to struggle with this (and still do). There were times when I'd be with my kids, feeling completely overstimulated, but I'd keep pushing through because I didn't want to inconvenience my wife, who, of course, was also carrying her share of parenting stress. I'd bottle it up, thinking I could handle it. But eventually, I'd hit a wall, and by then, I wasn't the parent or partner I wanted to be.

Speaking up and asking for help before I reach a breaking point is one of the most respectful things I can do for my family.

So speak up. Trust your partner. Honor your limits. When you ask for help, you're not stepping back from the team; you're leaning into it because no one wins by pretending to be invincible.

Teamwork in parenting isn't about getting everything right. It's about learning how to move in rhythm with your partner; sometimes leading, sometimes following, sometimes just catching your breath together in the background. The real strength of a partnership shows not in perfection, but in presence. In the way you carry the load together, even when it's heavy.

In James Norbury's moving book *Big Panda and Tiny Dragon*, there's a moment of quiet wisdom that speaks directly to this kind of partnership.

> *Which is more important. . .the journey or the destination? "The company," said Tiny Dragon," and "No matter how hard it gets," said Tiny Dragon, "we'll face it together," as said by Big Panda.*[2]

That's the core of what real partnership is, not splitting everything 50/50, not keeping score, but standing beside each other through the mess, the beauty, and the unknown. That's what you're building: not a perfect system, but a resilient one.

And if all else fails, just remember Chris Rock's wisdom: "Play that tambourine right." Show up. Keep the rhythm. And know that being a steady presence is just as important as taking the lead.

That's the energy to bring into your parenting: Unity. Strength. Love in motion.

In the next chapter, we'll explore the quieter magic: the small, everyday moments that often get lost in the noise. Because sometimes, what keeps a relationship strong isn't just surviving the hard parts; it's noticing the good ones. It's about those micro-moments of happiness, love, laughter, and stillness that remind you why you're doing this together in the first place that help relationships thrive.

Notes

1. *Chris Rock: Tambourine*, Netflix, 14 Feb 2018.
2. James Norbury, *Big Panda and Tiny Dragon* (Mandala Publishing, 2021).

11

The Secret Life of Small Moments

"Life's a journey, not a destination, and I just can't tell what tomorrow brings."
—Aerosmith ("Amazing")

MORE THAN TWO decades ago, I sat at a weekend retreat surrounded by friends when a speaker named Charlie Harary shared a story that has stayed with me ever since.

He told of a small town with a unique tradition: when children turned 13, they embarked on a journey to mark their transition into adulthood. For generations, everyone had chosen the path to the left, a road that led to relaxation, joy, and comfort. Along the way, they experienced tropical villas, calm beaches, and peaceful serenity. It was, by all accounts, a beautiful escape.

But one boy, known for his curiosity and adventurous spirit, wondered what lay down the path to the right. Against tradition, he chose it.

When he returned, the town eagerly gathered to hear his story. He didn't come back glowing or refreshed. He came back changed.

He explained that the first stop on the right path was a struggling farm. The work was grueling, the hours long, and his body ached. But over time, he saw the land come to life under his hands. What once felt like suffering transformed into purpose.

The second stop was a beach, not blissful, but polluted and dying. Garbage littered the shoreline, animals struggled to survive, and the stench was overwhelming. He spent weeks cleaning it, restoring it. When the beach finally sparkled again, the joy it brought the local community was indescribable.

The final stop was a small home, where an elderly couple was living out their final days. He cared for them, listened to their stories, and held space for their final moments. It was, he said, the most meaningful experience of his life.

The town was stunned. One person asked, "Why would anyone choose that path?" They couldn't comprehend why someone would willingly choose discomfort and difficulty.

But that young man had discovered something many overlook: true growth doesn't come from comfort. It comes from effort, presence, and the willingness to see value in the quiet, unnoticed parts of life. He saw the power in hard work, the beauty in service, and the depth in small, everyday moments.

The Myth of the "Perfect Moment"

In today's world, it's easy to get caught up in the idea that everything should be fun, exciting, and Instagram-worthy. We're bombarded with images of perfect families having perfect moments, and somehow everyone is smiling, and the kids well-behaved, not a hair out of place. We scroll through highlight reels and begin to wonder: why doesn't my life look like that?

The real danger isn't just the comparison. It's the subtle message that only picture-worthy moments are worth noticing. We lose sight of the value in the small, gritty, unpolished parts of life. We've forgotten that those sleepless nights and exhausting days have meaning. Parenting isn't just about the fun moments; it's about the effort we put in when no one is watching, the countless hours of work that often go unnoticed. It's about seeing the value in our hands-on approach, even when it feels like all we're doing is cleaning up messes and solving one crisis after another.

Some of the most transformative moments in parenting don't feel like breakthroughs at all. They feel exhausted. Frustration. Repetition.

Take sleep training or potty training, two of the most gloriously unglamorous tasks in the parenting world. In the thick of it, when you're on night seven of sleep deprivation or dealing with yet another accident, it's easy to question why you're putting yourself through it.

But then, one day, it clicks. Your child finally sleeps through the night or finally masters the potty, and in that moment, you realize all those hard days were leading to this. There's a sense of pride, a feeling of accomplishment that's hard to describe, but so incredibly satisfying. It's the realization that your efforts, no matter how grueling, actually mattered.

Parenting and our relationship with our partners and kids is about the power in the moments of our lives. The magic lives in the smallest of interactions: the belly laugh during bath time, the way your child's hand instinctively finds yours, the sleepy "I love you" whispered from the backseat. So many of us are hoping for the big moments that are "life-changing," but what we don't realize is that the smaller glimmers of everyday life change us in ways we don't recognize. All we have to do is pay attention.

Sonja Lyubomirsky says so powerfully in her book on happiness, "We habitually fail to enjoy, savor, and live in the present, as our minds are often someplace else. However, when you think about it, the present moment is all we are really guaranteed."[1]

Parenting is often about finding beauty in the mundane. It's about recognizing that the small, seemingly insignificant moments are what truly shape our relationships with our kids and partners.

Those spontaneous kisses from your child, the knowing look your partner gives you across a chaotic room, the softness of a hand on your back after a long day, or the quiet moments after they've finally fallen asleep in your arms, and you look down in awe that this bundle of cuteness is yours. These are the moments that fill your heart in ways you couldn't have imagined before becoming a parent.

We don't need more big moments. We need better attention to the small ones.

Activity #1: The Jar

Years ago, for our first anniversary, I did something simple that, in hindsight, I wish I had turned into a tradition.

I took a mason jar, grabbed some sticky notes, and started jotting down the small but meaningful moments we'd shared, funny things we said, small gestures of kindness, tiny everyday memories that made me pause with gratitude. By the end, the jar was filled with these simple, beautiful reminders of the life we were building.

Here's how it works:

Find a large jar or container, and keep a stack of sticky notes or index cards nearby. Throughout the year, anytime something small but meaningful happens, something that makes you laugh, cry, or feel, write it down and drop it in the jar.

It could be a sweet moment with your child, a loving glance from your partner, a milestone, a joke, or even a quote from a movie, TV show, or book that resonated with you that year. Anything that made an imprint. Anything you want to remember. Anything that makes you pause, smile, or feel.

Over time, the jar fills. And when it does, you'll be surprised at how much beauty you've forgotten. At the end of the year, take time to read through the notes. Reflect. Laugh. Cry. Feel grateful. Then start a new one.

You'll begin to see your life not just as a series of exhausting days but as a collection of meaningful, fleeting, powerful moments that deserve to be remembered.

Not long ago, I made a conscious effort to slow down and be more present with my wife and kids. I wanted to be more aware of these powerful moments that seem so minuscule to the outside.

Here's what I started to see:

- My kids snuggled up with my wife at bedtime, cozy in their pajamas, completely content.
- My children were laughing wildly on the trampoline, lost in a world where nothing else mattered.
- My daughter sitting quietly in a corner, reading to herself and then, sweetly, to her younger brother.
- The joy I feel every time I watch my wife playing with our kids, her laughter, her warmth, the simplicity of their connection.
- My son softly whispers, "I love you," greeting me with a playful "Hi, Mr. Sir," or smirking before gently licking my arm and tickling me.
- The look of love and understanding my wife and I share without saying a word.
- My grandmother sitting peacefully with my children, bridging generations in a moment of quiet wonder.
- My son falling asleep in my arms, his face calm and perfect, frozen in time.
- My wife reading in bed, our puppy curled up next to her—just a calm, content life at home.
- Sitting on the couch with my daughter, giggling, joking, and being utterly silly together.

None of these moments was staged or planned. They weren't big or flashy. But they mattered. And the more I noticed them, the more grounded I felt.

It is something so easy and accessible for all of us to do, allowing us to recognize the beauty and magic in our lives.

Screens Down, Hearts Open

A couple of months ago, I came across a quote that stopped me in my tracks:

"With our phones, we are forever elsewhere."

Sociologist Sherry Turkle coined this powerful insight, and Jonathan Haidt highlighted it further in his book *The Anxious Generation*. The truth of it hit me immediately.

How often have we found ourselves physically present yet emotionally and mentally miles away, buried deep in our screens, while life is unfolding around us?

Technology has quietly become our go-to escape route. Feeling bored? Reach for your phone. Awkward silence during dinner? Phone. A little anxious or uncomfortable? You know the drill, phone again. We're constantly teleporting ourselves into a digital world filled with curated highlights and endless scrolling, bypassing reality whenever it feels too messy or challenging. It feels harmless in the moment, but truthfully, each glance at our screens represents an active choice to avoid being fully present.

And I'm not preaching from some tech-free pedestal here, I'm just as guilty as anyone else. But lately, I've become increasingly aware of how my phone subtly interferes with my ability to connect deeply with those around me. I've caught myself scrolling Instagram while sitting next to my kids, checking emails during family time, half-listening while pretending to multitask.

The harsh reality is that this digital distraction slowly chips away at genuine happiness and authentic relationships. We're trading real laughter, love, and connection for pixels and pretend. Instead of truly experiencing life's moments, we're busy watching someone else's highlights, comparing, and craving validation through likes and follows. But genuine joy can't thrive in split attention; it demands our full, unfiltered presence.

This isn't a call to toss out technology entirely. Phones can be helpful, entertaining, and even connective. But we need to be honest with ourselves about the cost of constant distraction. Our screens should enhance our lives, not replace them.

So here's the honest, uncomfortable question we each need to ask:

> Is my relationship with technology pulling me closer to the people I love or quietly pushing me away?

Presence isn't a grand gesture. It's a choice. And the more we practice it, the more we notice what we've been missing all along.

When my daughter was about four, she was deep into this phase where she'd play "mom" to her stuffed animals. She'd line them up, talk to them, tuck them in, and give them all kinds of love, exactly the kind of stuff she sees from us. It was the cutest thing. But instead of jumping in or just being fully there with her, I was half-checked out, glued to my phone, probably answering emails or doing something that felt important in the moment.

And then, without warning, she walked over, grabbed the phone out of my hand, and said, "Daddy, you're missing all the fun! I can't raise these kids all by myself!" as she pointed to a pile of stuffed animals she'd just "given birth to."

I laughed because it was hilarious. She was right! I was missing it. I was missing her, this tiny, brilliant, creative moment she wanted to share with me. And for what? A to-do list? Some notification that could've waited?

That's the kind of moment you can't schedule. You can't re-create it. Either you show up for it or you don't.

I wasn't overcome with guilt, but I did feel a deep sense of regret. Not the kind that leads to shame, but the kind that makes you pause and ask: what matters right now?

That tiny, ridiculous scene, my daughter pretending to be a mom to her babies, wasn't just play. It was a connection, and I almost missed it.

Life is busy, phones are addicting, and we've all got way too much on our plates. But that moment reminded me that *presence is a choice.* I'd like to choose it more often. Because childhood is fast, memories are fragile, and those silly, tiny moments? They're everything.

That moment with my daughter reminded me how easy it is to miss what matters most, simply because we're distracted. And if I'm being honest, the hardest part isn't knowing that I need to be more present. It's figuring out how to do it in the middle of real life, busy, loud, overstimulating, and full of responsibilities.

So instead of trying to be perfect, I've started focusing on something else: being intentional—just one small shift at a time.

Activity: Let's Start Small

If you want to be more present, don't start with a massive lifestyle overhaul. Start small. Subtle shifts often have the biggest impact.

Step 1: Set a Tech-Free Boundary
Pick one moment in your day, just one, and make it sacred. For us, it's dinner. My wife and I agreed: no phones at the table. We leave them in the kitchen or on the counter so we can see and hear each other.

Step 2: Check In with Your Partner
Ask each other a hard but loving question:
  Are there moments when I feel like we're missing each other?
  This isn't about blame. It's about creating space to reconnect in the spaces where distraction has crept in. Maybe it's the end of the night on opposite ends of the couch, each on a screen. What if, instead, you spent 15 minutes talking? Sitting closer and sharing the day, just being there.

Step 3: Catch Yourself Drifting
When you feel that automatic scroll reflex, pause. Look up. Ask yourself: Is this where I want my attention right now?

Presence doesn't demand perfection. It requires practice.

Because life isn't happening on a screen, it's happening right in front of you. On your couch, at your dinner table, in the backseat of your car, in the beautiful in-between moments. And you deserve to be there for it.

Mini Moves, Major Impact

It's not unusual for clients to say, especially from women in long-term relationships, that it is a quiet, heartbreaking reflection:

> "We used to be so connected. We did little things for each other. We showed we cared. *What happened?*"

It's rarely said with anger. It's said with longing. When those small gestures start to disappear, it's never *just* about the gestures; it's about what they represent. The decline of playfulness and thoughtfulness, those little "I see you" moments, are warning lights, saying, "Hey, something deeper is going on."

There's this meme that floats around about wives noticing when their husbands stop smacking their tushy on the way by, and while it gets a laugh, there's truth buried in the humor. Those small moments of physical playfulness weren't just about flirtation. They said, "I see you. I'm thinking about you. I'm still into you." When it stops, people notice. And what they're wondering is, *Are we okay?*

Here's the good news: reconnecting doesn't require a massive overhaul or a dramatic gesture. You don't need a five-step intimacy plan or an over-the-top date night. I tell clients: **Think small. Be simple**. Think consistently. Love doesn't have to be loud or complicated. It just has to be *present*.

Here are a few real-life, low-effort, high-impact ideas I often suggest to couples:

- Create a secret handshake. It's dorky and goofy and totally yours. I have one with my daughter and wife; it connects us instantly.
- Give a quick kiss or a hug when you pass each other in the hallway. No buildup, just warmth.
- Reach out and touch your partner; a gentle hand squeeze, a soft arm graze, or a warm hug.
- Send a random "thinking of you" or "I love you" text. Or slip a sticky note into their bag or lunch.

- Use your ridiculous nicknames. Even the cringey ones. Especially the cringey ones. They say, "We have a thing." (Ours are Booger and Passion Fruit.)
- Make them a cup of coffee. Prep their meal. Toss in their favorite snack: small kindness, big ripple.

These aren't grand gestures. They're mini moves that carry weight, especially when done consistently. They say, "I haven't stopped choosing you."

This line from the book *The How of Happiness* drives it home: "Enjoy the little things, for one day you may look back and realize they were the big things."[2]

So instead of waiting for the perfect date night or a big reset, ask yourself:

What's one small thing I can do today to show up with love?

Then do it again tomorrow.

When I was a kid, one of my favorite places in the world was my grandparents' house—Omi and Opa, as I lovingly called them. Their home wasn't just a house; it was a haven filled with warmth, laughter, and a deep sense of belonging. It was a place where stories lived in every corner, and love was felt in every hug, every shared meal, every quiet moment.

One of my most vivid memories is sitting in a cozy side room with my mom and Oma, flipping through photo albums for hours. The room had this distinct smell and a shaggy rug I can still feel under my fingers. We'd look through old pictures, some filled with familiar faces, others of relatives I never had the chance to meet, but each one told a story, a thread in the larger tapestry of our family history.

Those afternoons were more than just strolls down memory lane. They were sacred moments. They were about connection. We weren't just looking at photos; we were remembering what mattered. I didn't fully understand it at the time, but I was learning something essential: that the shape of a life is found in the small, unassuming moments. Now, as a parent, I find myself re-creating that same experience with my kids. My wife has this beautiful habit of making a Shutterfly photo book every year. She gathers images from our phones and captures everything, from significant milestones like birthdays and vacations to the tiny, forgettable moments that end up meaning the most.

These books give us a chance to slow down and take it all in. We'll sit with our kids and flip through the pages, laughing, reminiscing, and sometimes tearing up. It's in those moments that we're reminded of just how meaningful our day-to-day life is.

To someone else, those pictures might look like just another birthday party or a random trip to the park, but to us, they're proof that joy and connection live in the everyday. They're evidence of a life well-loved. They hold the story of our family. Just like those afternoons with my grandparents shaped me, these moments help shape my children. They see themselves as part of something lasting. They see that their story matters.

As Robert Frost put it so poignantly: "Live life like it's the last breath you take, for that breath is the whole essence of living, the little things in life are what connects us to all the big things we live for."

Most of life won't feel like a highlight reel. It'll feel like laundry, bedtime routines, half-finished conversations, and moments that pass so quickly you almost miss them. But when you slow down and pay attention, you start to realize—those are the moments that matter most.

Because when we look back, it won't be the big vacations or picture-perfect days that stick with us. It'll be the small stuff: the quiet "I love yous," the way your partner reaches for your hand without thinking, the sound of your kids laughing in the other room. That's the good stuff. That's what we hold onto.

These moments are what keep us connected. They're what create the space for intimacy, for deeper connection, for finding our way back to each other.

In the next chapter, we will discuss intimacy. Not just physical but emotional too. The kind that makes you feel seen again. Heard again. Wanted again. Because sometimes, before we rebuild the spark, we have to slow down long enough to remember what brought us together in the first place.

Notes

1. Sonja Lyubomirsky, *The How of Happiness: A Scientific Approach to Getting the Life You Want* (Penguin Press, 2007).
2. ibid.

12

Rediscovering Us: More Than Just Date Night

"When you realize you want to spend the rest of your life with somebody, you want the rest of your life to start as soon as possible."
—Billy Crystal in *When Harry Met Sally*

Welcome to the world of parenthood and marriage, where maintaining a strong, intimate connection with your partner can feel like trying to find a matching pair of socks in a laundry basket full of chaos. Remember those pre-kid days, when your biggest dilemma was choosing between a nap, a Netflix binge, or maybe sneaking away for a spontaneous weekend trip?

Fast-forward to now: you're elbow-deep in diapers, snack negotiations, school forms, and the daily effort to keep everyone fed, clothed, and relatively sane. Finding time for connection with your partner can feel like trying to find a matching pair of socks in a laundry basket full of chaos.

When you're deep in the trenches of parenthood, finding time for each other can feel like a luxury you just can't afford or even consider due to all the responsibilities and required daily brain power.

Your relationship isn't just some side project you get to when the kids are asleep or when life slows down. Nurturing your relationship isn't a luxury; it's the foundation. It's the glue that holds everything else together. When that bond is strong, everything flows more smoothly: your parenting, your communication, your mental health. And when it's fraying? You feel it everywhere.

This chapter isn't about bringing back the honeymoon phase or pretending like kids didn't change things. It's about rediscovering the connection that made you choose each other in the first place. It's about making the daily choice to prioritize *your relationship*, not just the parenting team, but the partnership underneath it all.

When I first started working as a therapist, I was doing sessions at a fast-paced clinic in Queens, New York, trying to keep my head above water. I was undertrained, overwhelmed, and running on little more than coffee, impostor syndrome, and survival instinct. Oh—and I had a newborn at home. It's no surprise that I ended up having a panic attack during that time. Everything felt like too much, and I didn't yet have the tools or language to process it all.

A lot of that season is a blur, but one client said something I'll never forget. She was a new mom too, trying to figure out how to be a parent and still feel like a person, let alone a partner. She looked at me and said:

> *I feel like all I am doing with my husband is downloading information between us and there is no heart or feelings, just information.*

I felt the weight of her words, not just as her therapist, but as someone in the same boat because I knew exactly what she meant. Did you pack the lunch? Who's got drop-off tomorrow? Don't forget the pediatrician. I'll do the dishes if you do bath time.

It becomes a never-ending relay race of responsibilities. You're talking constantly—but you're not connecting.

And you're not doing anything wrong. You're managing a household, raising little humans, and trying to get through the day without forgetting to shower. But over time, if all your conversations are logistical updates, it chips away at your emotional bond.

You stop sharing feelings. You stop asking each other how you're really doing. The intimacy gets drowned out by the noise.

This is the subtle shift that happens to so many couples, not because they've fallen out of love but because life got loud. And if you don't catch it, you wake up one day realizing that you're roommates running a daycare instead of partners building a life.

When you invest in your relationship, you're not just showing up for your partner—you're showing up for yourself, too. You're building a space where you can both exhale. A space to feel seen, heard, and supported. A place where you're reminded that you're in this together, even when everything else feels like it's pulling you apart. And when that connection is nurtured, something shifts. You feel steadier. You communicate with more care. You recover from tension faster. It's not because life gets easier; it's because you're not carrying it all alone.

This isn't about putting more pressure on yourself to "fix" your marriage or make every night feel like a rom-com. It's about choosing to protect the bond that started it all. Not just for your partner. Not just for the kids. But because you deserve a relationship that restores you, not one that just survives the chaos.

Connection is the fuel. Not the reward after everything is done, but the thing that helps you keep going.

Beyond the Bedroom: What Intimacy Really Means Now

So how do you keep the spark alive when you're knee-deep in diapers, dishes, and the mental load of parenting? It starts with one shift: stop chasing perfect moments—and start creating intentional ones.

Date nights are great, but they're not the only way to reconnect. When people hear "date night," they often picture something elaborate: dinner reservations, babysitters, maybe an outfit without spit-up. But the truth is, it doesn't need to be fancy. It just needs to be *intentional*.

A shared laugh over a pint of ice cream.

A quick coffee together before the kids wake up.

A glass of wine on the porch after bedtime.

These are the small, quiet ways we say: *I still see you.*

I always think of this family I grew up with back in Long Island—my best friend's parents. They walked together every single day. Rain, snow, heatwave, you name it, they were out there. I used to call them the Post Office because they never skipped a day. That walk wasn't about exercise. It was about connection. It was their carved-out space to talk, vent, laugh, and just *be* together without the background noise of five kids.

The key is this: whatever connection looks like for you, make it non-negotiable. Put it on the calendar like you would a dentist appointment or a school event. You wouldn't cancel those, so don't cancel each other.

Let's be real—by the time the kids are in bed, you might feel more like collapsing than connecting. You're not alone. Most parents don't end the day thinking, *You know what sounds great right now? Effort.*

But here's a little secret: you don't have to go all out to make it special. Sometimes, the most romantic moments are the simplest. It could be as easy as cooking dinner together after the kids go to bed, lighting a few candles, and pretending you're in a fancy restaurant, even if you're just in your kitchen. The point is to focus on each other, even if it's just for a short while.

For my wife and me, it's board games. Monopoly Deal, Rummikub, or cards, whatever we can squeeze in. It's light, it's playful, and she absolutely destroys me. (Seriously, I think the win-loss record is something like 927–28.) But it's not about winning. It's about carving out time to laugh, compete, and just *be* together outside all the adulting.

You don't have to be in the mood for intimacy to create it. You just need to create a space where it can happen.

Start with this mantra: *Connection before perfection. Presence before pressure.*

Activity: Couples Journal

One thing I often recommend to couples, something my wife and I use ourselves, is what I call the "Just Thinking of You" journal.

Now, before you roll your eyes at the word "journal," hear me out. This isn't some emotional homework assignment. It's a shared notebook that lives on a nightstand or dresser filled with small, meaningful reminders that say: I see you, I'm thinking of you, and we matter.

You can write:

- *A funny story from your day*
- *A sweet memory that popped into your mind*
- *A little love note or inside joke*
- *A message of encouragement*
- *A quick "Thank you for doing bedtime last night."*

There are no rules, only intention. It's a gentle way to stay emotionally connected, especially during busy seasons when actual conversations feel hard to come by.

Now, if you're thinking, "What if I want to say something a little deeper?" that's valid too. Some couples choose to use this journal as a safe place to express frustrations or discuss moments of tension, especially when face-to-face conversations feel too charged or rushed.

That can work, but it requires a mutual agreement. You both have to set clear rules of engagement:

☑ *This space is for connection, not attack.*
☑ *Tone matters: stay kind, stay curious.*
☑ *Readiness to listen and repair should follow.*

Whether it's lighthearted or emotionally honest, the key is that this journal becomes a space for presence, not pressure. A way to say "We're still in this together" even when life is moving fast.

A few years ago, I was working with a dad who came into session feeling completely disconnected from his wife. He told me, "We're civil. We're functioning. But it's like we're coworkers raising a family, not a couple."

He wasn't angry. Just tired. Numb. He didn't know where to start.

So I asked him, "When's the last time you thanked her? Not for something big—just. . .anything?"

He paused. "I mean, I'm grateful. But I guess I haven't really said it in a while."

We talked about what it would be like to say "thank you" for the small stuff:

- Driving the kids to school
- Doing the dishes
- Folding the laundry
- Cleaning up after yourself
- Making dinner
- Putting the kids to bed
- Flushing the toilet
- (Insert daily thing here)

He thought it sounded too simple to matter. But he tried it anyway.

A few weeks later, he told me, "I started saying thank you every day. And now she's doing it back. Weirdly, our whole tone has changed. We're still exhausted. But we're gentler with each other."

It wasn't therapy breakthroughs or dramatic declarations. It was two words: *thank you.*

These small acts of appreciation help remind each other that you're still in this together, even when life gets hectic. Every small gesture says: I still choose you, and I still like you.

It's normal to feel guilty or even overwhelmed when you're not constantly focused on your kids and family. It's not about avoiding your role as a parent. It's about making space for your relationship, too, because when that connection is strong, everyone in the family benefits.

Keeping your relationship strong through parenthood isn't about grand gestures; it's about showing up with intention, creativity, and compassion for each other. The love might look different now, but it's no less real or worth fighting for. With a little effort, the spark can still glow—maybe not in the same way, but in a deeper, more lasting form. Because when you find each other in the middle of the noise, you remember: this is the bond that holds everything else together.

Lauren Smith Brody says it best: "Your marriage is the easiest relationship in the house to ignore."[1]

The most encouraging thing I've learned over the last 10 years of working with more than 100 couples is this:

Spending more than one hour alone a day makes a real difference.

The couples who managed to spend five hours or more together each week felt even more connected, sure, but what stood out was that anything over an hour showed a significant improvement in relationship satisfaction.

Now here's the catch: most couples only manage 20–35 minutes of real, uninterrupted time together per day. And in today's world of never-ending to-do lists and constant digital distractions, even that can feel ambitious.

But one to three hours a week? With some planning and intention, that's within reach. And it can change everything.

To keep that love alive (or at least from flatlining during the harder seasons), here are three key mindsets to hold onto:

1. Don't aim so high.
2. This is temporary.
3. Keep trying.

Don't Aim So High

I've lost count of how many couples have said, "But I don't want to *settle*." I get it. No one wants to feel like they're giving up on passion or connection. But adjusting your expectations doesn't mean lowering your standards; it means *updating them* to fit your current reality.

Recently, a couple told me, "We're just not who we were when we were dating."

My response? *Good. You're not supposed to be.*

Life has changed, so your relationship needs to evolve with it. If you hold your connection today up to the glow of a different season (pre-kids, more sleep, fewer demands), you'll constantly feel disappointed. Not because your relationship is broken but because you're comparing it to a version that no longer fits.

If your standards are sky-high and completely unrealistic, of course you're going to feel disappointed and unloved. You'll feel let down, not because the love is gone but because you're measuring it by the wrong standards. The goal isn't to go backward. It's about building something new together at this stage.

This Is Temporary

When you're in the thick of stress, disconnection, or exhaustion, it can feel like this is just how life will be forever. That hopeless feeling? Totally valid. But it's also shortsighted.

When we examine our scenarios, we must be honest about what we can do and what we know in our hearts and accept that this is a *now issue*, not a *forever struggle*.

Life is always moving and progressing, whether we want it to or not, but we need to learn to accept what it brings us today.

If there is an opportunity, take it! If one weekend the grandparents or family take the kids for a few hours, say yes and jump for joy. But don't sulk in the thought that it happens only occasionally, because there will be a time when you can do more, be more, and connect in the way you wished when the kids were little. It will happen when the kids don't need you as much, and then you'll wish they were around more to need you.

There will always be a "grass is greener" mentality about other couples and their situations. Stop grading yourself on someone else's edited version. Their situation is not yours. Their pace is not yours. So put the phone down. Stop scrolling. Start noticing what your life is offering *today* and how you can show up for each other in the small but meaningful ways that count.

Don't Stop Trying

Of everything I've shared, this matters most: Don't stop trying. Ever.

Keep coming back to each other. Keep testing ideas. Keep tossing out what doesn't work and doubling down on what does. You can't coast your way to closeness—relationships don't run on cruise control. They need regular, intentional fuel to keep going.

The moment you stop trying, stop initiating, stop noticing, stop caring, is the moment your relationship starts to quietly fade. You don't become enemies. You become roommates, co-existing but no longer connecting.

All that love you built, all the memories, the effort, the inside jokes, it deserves to keep growing. And that means choosing, again and again, to keep showing up. To not give up.

Because trying is loving, and loving, especially in the middle of parenting chaos, is the bravest thing you can do.

Activity: Baseline Love

This activity is about identifying and protecting the *baseline expressions of love* that help you feel grounded in your relationship, even when time and energy are limited. We all have things we do or say that prove to us that our relationship is good, loving, and doing well.

Sit down together and talk through this question:

What are the small things—daily or weekly—that make you feel loved, appreciated, and connected?

Think of them as the minimum effort needed to keep the emotional pilot light on, even in survival mode.

Here are a few examples:

- A daily check-in text just to say "thinking of you"
- A kiss goodbye in the morning, no matter how rushed
- Saying "thank you" for routine things like dishes or bedtime

(continued)

(*continued*)

- Sending a funny meme that made you laugh
- A ritual bedtime phrase or inside joke

In my marriage, we say the same line before bed every night: **"Sleep well. Dream big. You are my something, you are my everything."**

No matter what happened that day, whether we fought, felt distant, or barely spoke, that phrase grounds us. It's our signal that love is still here, that we're still choosing each other.

Tip: Write down three to five baseline rituals or expressions that work for you. Post them somewhere visible or keep them in a shared note. They should feel doable, meaningful, and personal, not performative.

From Touched Out to Turned On

As a couples therapist, I go everywhere with my clients—from parenting chaos to emotional ruts, and yes, right into the bedroom. It's not just about sex for the sake of sex. It's about what it *represents*: emotional safety, closeness, being seen, and feeling wanted.

I can't tell you how many couples walk into my office saying they're "not connecting physically," but what they're telling me is: *We've stopped feeling like us.*

I still remember a client telling me:

"The emotional connection is what warms the oven for physical connection."

Emotional intimacy isn't separate from physical intimacy; they feed into each other. When you feel emotionally safe, understood, and appreciated, you're far more likely to want to open up physically. However, when one of those pieces is ignored or neglected, the entire system begins to suffer. If you stop actively working on one, you can expect the other to slow down or even shut down entirely.

Being touched out is real. After a long day of wiping noses, managing tantrums, juggling work, and giving all of yourself to your kids, the last thing many parents want is one more person needing something from them, even if it's their partner. But here's where small, consistent gestures matter. It's not always about being ready for sex—it's about staying connected *so* the door to intimacy stays open.

Start with playfulness:

- A spontaneous hug in the kitchen
- A wink across the room
- A text that says, "Can't stop thinking about you"
- Or just lying next to each other without distractions

Don't stop kissing. Don't stop flirting. Don't stop touching *without expectation*. These are the building blocks of trust and connection that allow physical intimacy to grow again, even after seasons of stress or disconnection.

And don't stop telling your partner how much you're still attracted to them. Not because it's a line or a duty, but because they deserve to know. Talk about what intimacy looks like now—not what it used to be, not what it "should" be—but what feels possible and meaningful today.

I once had a client say, "We're not in the honeymoon phase anymore, and that makes me sad." And I get that. But I reminded them, *the honeymoon is about sparks. Long-term love is about warmth.* It's steadier, deeper, and more sustaining. . .but only if you keep showing up for it.

As Van Gogh once said, "I feel that there is nothing more truly artistic than to love people."

Love, especially in parenthood, is an art, a skill, and a daily practice.

You might not be all over each other like in your twenties—but that doesn't mean the heat is gone. It just might look like a long hug at the end of a hard day. A slow dance in the kitchen. Or a quiet moment where you look at each other and know: *we're still us.*

So much shifts when you become parents—your identity, your routines, your energy, your relationship. What used to come so naturally might now feel like one more thing to figure out. But just because it takes more effort doesn't mean the connection is gone. It's still there, under the noise and exhaustion. Under the schedules and the to-do lists. You just have to find your way back to it—together.

It's easy to think intimacy means grand gestures or weekly date nights (and hey, if you can swing those, great). But the real stuff? It's often quiet. A glance that says "We've got this." A sleepy thank you. A smirk across the room when your kid says something absurd. That's the love that keeps you going.

If you're not feeling that right now, it doesn't mean you're doing anything wrong. It means you're human. And parenting is a full-contact, full-time, emotionally relentless experience. Disconnection doesn't mean your relationship is broken—it just means it's time to check in. Maybe slow down. Maybe reach for each other in small ways again.

And if part of what's been lost is you, who you are outside of being a parent, that's okay too. You matter—your desires, your needs, your sense of self. When you reconnect with that part of you, it brings more depth and energy into your relationship too.

So maybe tonight, just say the thing you've been holding back. A compliment. A memory. A "Thanks for doing bedtime; I know you're exhausted too." Maybe it's a quick kiss on the forehead or a hand on their back as you pass in the hallway. Tiny moments add up. You don't need fireworks to prove you still love each other. You just need a spark and a reason to notice it.

Because in the end, your relationship isn't just a side project. It's the heartbeat of your family and the foundation you both stand on.

And that spark? It's not gone. It's just waiting for you to notice it again.

Intimacy isn't just about sex—it's about knowing and being known. It's built in the way you listen, the way you touch, the way you choose to see each other when life makes it easy to look away.

It will change over time. It should. But change doesn't have to mean loss—it can mean depth, resilience, and a kind of closeness that outlasts the rush of the early days.

If there's one truth to carry forward, it's this: intimacy doesn't happen by accident. You create it. You protect it. You keep showing up for it, even when it feels inconvenient, awkward, or vulnerable.

Because the couples who last aren't the ones who never struggle—they're the ones who never stop reaching for each other. And the ones who keep their connection? They're not the ones who never drift—they're the ones who always find their way back.

Drifting happens. Staying lost is optional.

Note

1. Lauren Smith Brody, *The Fifth Trimester: The Working Mom's Guide to Style, Sanity, and Success After Baby* (National Geographic Books, 2018).

Conclusion

"The best and most beautiful things in the world cannot be seen or even touched. They must be felt with the heart."

—Helen Keller

Never Say I Can't

When I was in third grade, I had one of the best teachers of my life: Mrs. Itzkowitz. She also happened to be my backyard neighbor growing up in Long Island. Bursting with energy, love, and kindness, she taught me how to read time, believe in myself, and embrace all the quirks and weirdness that make us beautifully human.

One of the most powerful memories I carry from her classroom has stayed with me to this day, and it's something I hope to pass on to my kids and you.

One morning, she had written a bunch of negative "I can't" statements on the board. They were all the ways kids talk themselves out of trying: "I can't do math," "I can't draw," "I can't be good at sports." She looked at us and said, "None of these belongs in my classroom. They're not welcome here because they stop us from growing."

She then had us do a project. We sat quietly and wrote out every "I can't" that came to mind. My list had things like:

I had things like:

- I can't do math.
- I can't write clearly (I still have terrible handwriting).
- I can't be an astronaut.
- I can't sing.
- I can't play basketball.
- I can't run fast.
- I can't do the monkey bars.
- I can't write good (remember, I was in third grade).
- I can't spell good.

And the list went on.

After that, we cut each statement into strips, placed them in a shoebox, and went outside to the grassy patch behind the school. One by one, we read our statements out loud, tossed them into the box, and buried them.

Then she said something that has echoed in my mind ever since:

"From this moment on, you're no longer the reason you don't achieve your goals. If something's hard, ask for help. Try again. Try differently. Never stop chasing greatness for yourself. But don't say you can't and limit yourself just because you haven't figured it out yet. You always can!"

That day, I felt unstoppable.

I'll be honest: one of the biggest "I can't" statements I've carried into adulthood is "I can't write." Whether it was a school paper, a blog post, or a tweet, I just didn't see myself as a "writer." So to be sitting here, wrapping up an actual book, is more than a career milestone. It's a personal victory. It's me burying that "I can't" in the ground, for good.

So, thank you! For reading this, for giving me the chance to prove myself wrong, and for reminding me that growth is always possible.

And now I want to ask you: What limiting beliefs are you still carrying? What invisible rule have you made for yourself or your relationship that's quietly whispering, "You're not enough"? I'm not saying that everything is possible just because we want it badly enough, but I am saying, *try*.

Try with all your heart. Ask for help. Seek out guidance. Use what you have. And don't give up before you've really started.

I've been asked a lot lately how this book came to be. The truth is, I just kept going. I started a podcast during COVID at a time when I, like so many others, felt totally ungrounded. Writing still scared me, so I started talking instead.

Since then, I've recorded more than 250 episodes, had conversations with incredible people, and built a network that has changed my life. One of my dream guests, Slumberkins, took me 2.5 years of pitching to finally get a yes. Why? Because I stopped saying "I can't" and started asking anyway.

That same interview led to a connection with Wiley Publishing. They heard my voice, sass and all, and offered me the chance to write a book about a topic that has shaped my personal life and professional passion.

I still can't quite believe it. But here we are.

If you found this book because you felt stuck, disconnected, or maybe even hopeless in your relationship, I want you to hear this clearly:

You *haven't* given up. You're here. You're looking for guidance, hope, and a way forward. That means you're still in it. That means you still care.

Trying doesn't always look like grand romantic gestures or epic breakthroughs. Sometimes trying looks like picking up a book, highlighting a passage, sending a text instead of going to bed angry, or reading one more chapter after the kids are asleep.

And that counts. That matters.

You are actively choosing your relationship. You are finding another way forward.

This book won't fix everything. But it's a guide for small, daily choices that can get you moving in the right direction, not back to where you were but forward to where you want to go.

It's not about perfect communication, constant passion, or having it all figured out. It's about being honest, doing your best with what you have, and believing that your relationship is still worth the effort.

So bury your own "I can't" statements.

Say:

I can love again.

I can show up differently.

I can try one more time.

I can ask for help.

I can grow.

You've made it to the end of this book, which means you've already done something many people avoid—you've looked your relationship in the eye and said, "You're worth the work." That's no small thing.

We began this journey in the chaos—the sleep-deprived, tension-filled, "Who even are we right now?" season of parenting. The truth is, some days, we're still there. But now, we know the map a little better. We've learned where the potholes are and how to slow down before we hit them.

My hope for you isn't a perfect road. It's the courage and tools to keep traveling it together. Parenting will keep changing you— let it. Let it deepen your love, sharpen your patience, and make you braver.

Here's my promise: there will be days when parenting feels impossible, nights when your relationship feels distant, and moments when you wonder if you're still the same people who said, "I do."

That's normal. But marriage doesn't stop at "I do." The real work—the real love—is in how you keep choosing "we do," day after day.

But it's also a reminder that your relationship is not a side project to raising kids—it's the foundation everything else rests on. Protect it. Feed it. Let it matter. Because when it's strong, you're strong. And strong couples make strong families.

Love in this season isn't effortless—it's built. Brick by brick. Choice by choice. Day after day. That's where the magic is.

And if you remember nothing else, remember this:

Don't stop trying, because YOU CAN.

Appendix

Import/Export

IN	OUT

Acknowledgments

I NEED TO first start with thanking G-d. If it weren't for my faith and belief, I wouldn't be in the place I am today. He has put in the right places, around the right people, and in the right situations to be successful in life. I owe everything to him.

To my wife, **Ariella**:

You are everything! Since I met you, I have been a better man every day of the last 11 years. Every day I challenge myself to be a true support for you, which has turned me into a more attuned man, a more vulnerable man, and a full feeling human. You have given me everything I ever need: love, support, and, of course, our amazing kids.

We have been through so much together and through the stress, late-night conversations, and joys of this journey of writing a book and of letting me be so honest and real about our own journey, you have let me be me, and that is one of the most powerful things you could have done for me to be the best person for you and the kids.

To my daughter **Rikki/Rikster/Pickle**:

You made me a father, something I have dreamed about since I was a teenager. You have taught me how to be softer, bringing out so much silliness and love I never knew I had in me. Thank you for keeping me grounded and focused over the years to push myself and drive for more, so you can have more. This book started because you came into our lives and taught us so much from day one, and I hope you continue to grow into the amazing woman I know you will become. Thank you for all the cuddles, laughs, and love you bring into my life. I love you!

To my son **Max/Pookie Pants/Little Dude**:

You pushed me more than anyone else. When you came along, I thought I had it all figured out. I was so confident with my parenting skills, and you immediately humbled me to open my mind and heart to learn and grow even more. You have created such a wackiness in our home and energy that means so much. You are such a yumball, and I love you so so much.

To my **parents**:

If it weren't for you, I would not be the man I am today. I wouldn't have been instilled with the values, life perspectives, and inner strength if it weren't for your support and guidance over the years. I'm sure sitting reading this (and me writing this), you can't believe I wrote a whole book! When I was younger, I truly struggled with school with all my ADHD struggles, and all you did was help, love, and find any way possible to get me through it all. Well, I made it through and beyond all because of you both. I never knew how much parents did for their kids until I became one, and I can never thank you enough for not killing me a long time ago, always being there, and providing all you could and all you sacrificed for me.

Thank you, **Abba**, for being the quiet calm in my life—the steady presence I can always turn to for advice, wisdom, and perspective. You don't need to be the loudest voice in the room (I've got that covered), because your strength comes through in consistency, integrity, and the way you show up. I genuinely trust you and look up to you—not just as a guiding force but as a living example of what it means to be a father who shows up with love, humility, and purpose.

Thank you, **Mommy**; you've shown me what it means to fully feel and to embrace all the wackiness and uniqueness of our personalities. As your twin, I've learned so much from your journey, from the challenges you've faced to the successes you've achieved. Thank you for always having my back and for being there through it all— the tears, the laughs, and the hugs that remind me I'm never alone.

To my **in-laws**:
Thank you for all the support you have given me and my family. You are always willing to help us when we need it, and especially through this process you have been such cheerleaders and babysitters to help me get through this adventure of writing a book. And more importantly you raised an amazing woman who has changed my life for the better. I never knew I could be loved by another set of parents close to the way my parents do, and y'all truly give me so much love.

Ma-Ma Siegs, thank you for being the kind of mother-in-law who drops everything for us and the kids without a second thought. Your selflessness, love, and steady presence have carried us through so many moments—big and small. Whether it's stepping in with the kids, supporting us when life feels overwhelming, or simply showing up with open arms, you've been our anchor. I'm endlessly grateful for the way you love us and for the example you set of generosity and devotion.

To **Pops**, thank you for your endless cheerleading, your constant smiles, and the love you pour into our family. The way you beam with pride, brag about me to others, and celebrate every step I take makes me feel so deeply seen and appreciated. Add to that your joyful spirit (and yes, your tears), and you've taught me that true strength isn't about holding back but about showing up with heart. You've proven that strong men cry—and it's not just me! I'm forever grateful for your love, your pride, and the way you've always lifted me up.

To my **Opa**:

Even though he passed away when I was just 13, my Opa has remained a guiding force in my life. Nearly every day, I find myself asking, *What would Opa do?* He was a powerhouse, someone who left a mark on everyone he met and poured his heart into everything he pursued. I owe so much of my inner drive, my relentless self-critic, and even a bit of my stubborn determination to him. He's the reason I keep pushing myself to show up, grow, and try to make the world around me just a little bit better every day.

To **Wiley Publishers/Jossey-Bass**:

Thank you, **Amy Fandrei**, you have truly been a therapist through this entire process. You have pushed me the right way, supported my spirals and doubts, and been there when I needed some kick-in-the-butt energy. I still can't believe this is happening, and the fact you gave me a chance and believed in me is one of the most powerful things you could have ever done for me.

Sophie Thompson, you have truly kept me on task and helped work out all the nitty-gritty of details, always being there when I need it.

Pete Gaughan, I always appreciate someone who says it like it is and directs me in an honest and true way. Thank you for being such a guiding force through this process and helping the book be an A+ for the readers. I know there was a lot of work that needed to be done.

To the rest of the team, all I did was put words on a page, but you took it to the next level to make it magical and reality. Thank you from every cell in my body that you helped a distant dream become a reality.

To **Dr. Stanley Rustin, Dr. Alan Perry, Jenna Tine, and Sally Oshinsky:**

If it weren't for you, I wouldn't be the therapist I am today. You shaped me with kindness, realness, and honesty of being a therapist. You answered every question, sat with me when I thought I couldn't do it, and listened through all the doubts, tears, and stress of the process of becoming a therapist. All my client's success is due to the lessons and leadership you gave me through the last 15 years.

To my **Fordham professors:**

Thank you for seeing me, challenging me, and believing in me even when I doubted myself. Your guidance shaped not only my career but also the person I strive to be. The lessons you taught, the encouragement you offered, and the way you modeled compassion and curiosity live on in every page of this book. I am forever grateful.

To all my **clients:**

This book wouldn't have happened if you hadn't embraced my style of therapy throughout the years. You have all taught me so much about being human and all the complexities life has for us. You have let me listen, learn, and grow with you throughout the 10 years. This book wouldn't have happened if you hadn't let me into your lives.

About the Author

ELI WEINSTEIN, is a licensed clinical therapist, podcast host, international speaker, and proud husband and father of two, based in Las Vegas. With a thriving private practice serving clients in both New York and Nevada, Eli is known for his refreshingly relatable approach to therapy, blending clinical expertise with warmth, authenticity, and a no-BS attitude. His work is rooted in helping people navigate the beautiful realities of relationships, parenting, mental health, and personal growth.

Eli is the creator and host of *The Dude Therapist* podcast, where for more than five years he's interviewed thought leaders and mental health and wellness experts in candid, down-to-earth conversations. His insights have been featured on *The Kelly Clarkson Show*, in *Psychology Today*, and across more than 300 podcast appearances, earning him a reputation for making emotional and relational topics feel accessible, human, and deeply resonant.

As the founder of **ELIvation**, Eli delivers impactful keynotes, workshops, and one-on-one coaching to individuals, couples, and organizations around the globe. Whether on stage or in session, he meets people where they are, combining therapeutic insight with real-world application to spark meaningful growth and connection.

In his debut book, *From I Do to We Do: Navigating Marriage Through Parenting Years* (Wiley, 2025), Eli dives into the often unspoken challenges couples face while raising children. Through humor, vulnerability, and clinical wisdom, he offers practical tools to help partners stay emotionally connected—even in the chaos.

Whether through therapy, podcasting, or public speaking, Eli's mission is clear: to help people grow, connect, and thrive—without losing themselves along the way.

If this book resonated with you; sparked a thought, a question, or just made you feel seen. I'd love to hear from you.

You can reach me at **eliweinsteinlcsw@gmail.com**, visit **www.eliweinsteinlcsw.com**, or find me on Instagram **@eliweinstein _lcsw**.

Your stories and reflections keep these conversations alive and remind me why I love doing this work and why none of us are ever truly alone in it.

Index

Note: Page number in **bold** refers to Active Tip, Activity and Tip.